SHAMANIC PLANT MEDICINE

San Pedro:
The Gateway
to Wisdom

Shamanic Plant Medicine

San Pedro:
The Gateway
to Wisdom

Ross Heaven

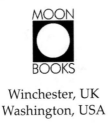

MOON
BOOKS

Winchester, UK
Washington, USA

First published by Moon Books, 2016
Moon Books is an imprint of John Hunt Publishing Ltd., Laurel House, Station Approach,
Alresford, Hants, SO24 9JH, UK
office1@jhpbooks.net
www.johnhuntpublishing.com
www.moon-books.net

For distributor details and how to order please visit the 'Ordering' section on our website.

Text copyright: Ross Heaven 2015

ISBN: 978 1 78279 255 0
Library of Congress Control Number: 2016934812

A CIP catalogue record for this book is available from the British Library.

Design: Stuart Davies

Printed and bound by CPI Group (UK) Ltd, Croydon, CR0 4YY, UK

We operate a distinctive and ethical publishing philosophy in all
areas of our business, from our global network of authors to
production and worldwide distribution.

CONTENTS

About the Author   vi

Introduction: Shamanic Plant Medicine   1
The First Practical Guide to Working with Teacher Plants

Chapter 1. The Story of Huachuma   4
'Those who drink its juice lose their senses and are as if dead.'
    An introduction to the history of San Pedro, its
    shamanic uses and contemporary work with the plant

Chapter 2. Healing with San Pedro   35
'Yes, Yes, Yes, You Are Going to be Cured.' Key themes and
    lessons that arise from shamanic work with San Pedro.
    How the plant conducts its healings, including new case
    studies of those who have been healed by it

Chapter 3. Cactus Creativity   86
'Learn to think outside of your head.' How San Pedro opens
    the heart and mind to greater creativity

Chapter 4. Working Responsibly with San Pedro   115
Advice on staying safe and getting the most from your
    work with huachuma

Appendix   130
A deeper explanation of some Andean healing concepts
    and terms

Endnotes   133

About the Author

Ross Heaven is a shaman and the author of several books on shamanism, plant teachers and healing and runs workshops on these themes in Europe and Peru, including Shamanic Apprenticeship training programs, Shamanic Healing and Soul Retrieval courses, as well as plant medicine retreats with San Pedro, salvia divinorum, mushrooms and ayahuasca, and journeys to Peru to work with indigenous shamans. He is also a therapist and provides counseling, soul retrieval and healing.

Ross has a website at www.thefourgates.org where you can read more about his work as well as forthcoming books and other items of interest. He also provides a monthly newsletter by email, which you can receive free of charge by contacting ross@thefourgates.org.

His other books on plant teachers and medicines include *Cactus of Mystery*, *The Hummingbird's Journey to God* and *Drinking the Four Winds* (three books about San Pedro), *Plant Spirit Shamanism* (about ayahuasca and Amazonian plant healing) and *The Sin Eater's Last Confessions* (about Celtic methods of soul healing with herbs and plants).

Other books by Ross in the Shamanic Plant Medicine series include *Ayahuasca*, *Salvia Divinorum* and *Sacred Mushrooms*. His full book list can be viewed at Amazon Books.

Introduction: Shamanic Plant Medicine

The First Practical Guides to Working with Teacher Plants

Shamanic Plant Medicine is a series of books written to provide you with a succinct and practical introduction to a specific teacher or power plant, its history, shamanic uses, healing applications and benefits, as well as the things to be aware of when working with these plants, including ceremonial procedures and safety precautions. These plants are also known in the Western world as entheogens: substances that 'reveal the God within', and in shamanic cultures as allies: helpful spirits that confer power and pass on insights and information.

The first in this series are *Ayahuasca: The Vine of Souls, San Pedro: The Gateway to Wisdom, Salvia Divinorum: The Sage of the Seers* and *Sacred Mushrooms: Messengers of the Stars*. It is a series that reveals the truth about these plants and provides an insight into their uses as well as the cautions to take with them so you are properly informed of your choices, not reliant on government propaganda, media sensationalism and disinformation. Then you can make your own decisions.

The shamanic use of plants and herbs is one of the world's oldest healing methods and, despite government and media campaigns to the contrary, it is usually the safest and most effective form of medicine too. In 2005, for example, the British Medical Journal warned that 'in England alone reactions to [legally available prescription] drugs that led to hospitalization followed by death are estimated at 5,700 a year and could actually be closer to 10,000.' By comparison, in the *four* years between 2000 and August 2004 there were just 451 reports of adverse reactions to herbal preparations and only 152 were considered serious. No fatalities. That statistic equates to just 38 problem cases a year resulting from plant medicines compared to perhaps 10,000 deaths a year as a result of accepted mainstream medicine. Reviewing these figures the London Independent newspaper concluded that: 'Herbs may not be completely safe as critics like to point out – but they are a lot safer than drugs.'

The situation in America is similar. Here, orthodox medical treatment itself is now the leading cause of death, ahead of heart disease and cancer, while: 'Infections, surgical mistakes and other medical harm contributes to the deaths of 180,000 hospital patients a year [and] another 1.4 million are seriously hurt by their hospital care.' (Consumer Reports online: www.consumer-reports.org.) Even more sobering is the fact revealed by other studies that adverse drug reactions are under-reported by up to 94 percent in the US since the government does not adequately track them. Deaths as a result of plant healings meanwhile remain next to zero, and they can be as effective – or more so – than prescription medications.

It is worth asking why these figures so often go unreported and why the medical profession continues to treat people as it does even with full awareness of the risks and comparisons. Another good question is why plants and herbs more than drugs and orthodox medicine are the focus of governments for stricter regulation (see for example the current *codex alimentarius* proposals) despite their effectiveness and comparative freedom from risk. Who benefits, especially financially, from this state of affairs?

More remarkable even than their ability to heal the body is the ability of some plants to expand the mind, raise consciousness, release stuck or damaging emotions and connect us more deeply to spirit. These are the teacher plants. By showing us our true power and potential they enable us to see through illusions and explore the real nature of the dreaming universe so we discover our purpose on Earth.

Plant teachers are used by shamans the world over in a sacred ritual context to divine the future, enter spirit realms, learn the deepest truths of themselves and the universe (although many shamans see little distinction between the two since, as they say, 'the world is as you dream it'; that is, each of us *is* the universe). They also enable them – and us – to perform true healings, which go beyond the abilities of modern medicine and its reliance on intrusive treatments and often damaging drugs.

There is a sort of mystery surrounding San Pedro and a sense that knowledge of the plant must remain secret or at least be earned through preparation, participation, and the worthiness of those who drink it.
Ross Heaven in *The Hummingbird's Journey to God* (O-Books 2009)

Chapter 1

The Story of Huachuma

'Those Who Drink its Juice Lose their Senses and are as if Dead'

The Spanish Inquisition reacted with characteristic savagery to anyone who dared to break their laws by eating [San Pedro]...a great many Indians were flogged and sometimes killed when they persisted

Jim DeKorne, writing about the history of San Pedro

San Pedro (*Trichocereus pachanoi*) is a tall blue-green cactus reaching heights of 23 feet (7m) or more. It enjoys a tough desert-like environment and grows readily in the highest parts of its native Peru, but can also be found in central and north America and in some Mediterranean countries. In most countries, including the UK, the cactus can be bought openly in garden centers as owning and growing it is not illegal, and even if the weather is not conducive to planting it out (countries like the UK, for example, are too wet and cold to sustain it), it will thrive as a house plant and is easily maintained, putting on maybe 12 inches to 18 inches in height a year if treated well.

Sitting in a plant pot or in a garden border at home, the plant looks attractive, innocent and innocuous. In terms of its spiritual, healing and consciousness-expanding properties, however, it is one of the most powerful teacher plants in the world. This contradiction between appearance and spiritual potency is one of the reasons why, in medicine circles, San Pedro has come to be known as the Cactus of Mystery.

It has other names too among the shamans and healers of the Peruvian Andes, including *cardo, chuma, gigantón, hermoso, huando, pene de Dios* (literally, 'penis of God'), *wachuma* and, simply, *el remedio*: the remedy, the latter referring to its healing powers. One of its Quechua names is *punku*, which means 'doorway' or 'gateway', since the cactus is also considered able to open a portal into a world beyond illusion so that healing and visions can flow from the spiritual to the physical dimension. Its more common name, San Pedro, has similar connotations. It refers to Saint Peter, who holds the keys to Heaven, and is suggestive of the plant's power to open the gates between the visible and invisible worlds so those who drink it enter a realm where they can heal, know their true natures and find purpose for their lives. Because of these protective and nurturing qualities, others refer to it affectionately as simply Papa or Grandfather.

The Hidden Keys to Heaven: San Pedro in Ancient Times

According to tradition, it was San Cipriano (Saint Cyprian), the patron saint of magicians, the grand exorcist, and the 'soul of the *mesa'* (the healing altar used during ceremonies by San Pedro shamans) who, acting on instructions from Jesus, hid the keys to Paradise within the cactus, under the care and guardianship of Saint Peter (San Pedro). The legend goes that God was so appalled at the behavior of the Spanish who invaded Peru in search of El Dorado (the fabled city of gold) and was so concerned that they might find these magical keys and use them to storm the gates of Heaven in search of greater riches that he had Cipriano hide them in the one place he knew the Catholic invaders would never look: inside a cactus that had been used as a pagan sacrament for centuries before the coming of the Catholics and Conquistadors.

The point of God's deception was that all seekers must earnestly desire to meet Him with open hearts and minds and in a reverent and dignified manner, and this is something that God did not see in the frenzied desire for gain, which drove the Spanish to destruction and murder. The cactus demanded purity: a return to a first state where true love and faith, not illusions or pretences at love to support an Earthly lust for gold, was the force that dictated their actions. This approach of open heart and mind and an attitude of earnest yet respectful desire for healing and enlightenment is still the requirement of the cactus for those who come seeking the blessings of San Pedro.

God's great deception worked too. When the Spanish began their invasion of the Incan empire from 1532 they brought with them their own understanding of God, a prissy, precious, church-bound angry desert God who would have no truck with or tolerance for the savage heathen rituals they witnessed among the natives. As a result of their own prejudice they completely missed the magic of the cactus and its relationship to the true God. Thus, one 16th century Conquistador described huachuma as a plant used by heathens to 'speak with the devil', while a Spanish missionary decried it as 'a plant with whose aid the devil is able to strengthen the Indians in their idolatry; those who drink its juice lose their senses and are as if dead; they are almost carried away by the drink and dream a thousand unusual things and believe that they are true'.

Rather than trying to understand native customs or explore the potential of huachuma to illuminate their own religion or bring healing and peace to the soul, these 'men of God', the Spanish Inquisition, 'reacted with characteristic savagery to anyone who dared to break their laws by eating it', according to Jim DeKorne in *Psychedelic Shamanism*.

A great many Indians were flogged and sometimes killed when they persisted in using [huachuma]... [One man's] eyeballs were said to be gouged out after three days of torture; then the Spaniards cut a crucifix pattern in his belly and turned ravenous dogs loose on his innards.[1]

Throughout all of this persecution, however, the natives never once gave up the secrets of the cactus and the knowledge of God it contained, preferring to be killed or to kill themselves, like the hero Quispe, than to betray the wishes of God. Through their sacrifices they ensured that huachuma remained the Cactus of Mystery.

Cactus Origins

The original name of San Pedro in Peru was *huachuma*, a Quechua word that simply means 'dizzy'. This is a reference to one of the effects of the cactus medicine and another indicator of the mystery surrounding this plant, since it gives no suggestion of the deeper and more profound spiritual and healing effects that are experienced when drinking it, and which are actually more common than dizziness. The shamans who worked with it were therefore called *huachumeros* if male or *huachumeras* if female. The earliest archaeological evidence so far discovered for its use as a sacrament in healing rituals is in the form of a stone carving of a huachumero found at the Jaguar Temple of Chavín de Huantar in northern Peru, which is about 3,500 years old, predating the birth of Christ. Textiles from the same region and period depict the cactus with jaguars and hummingbirds, its guardian spirits, and with stylized spirals representing the visionary experiences given by the plant. A decorated ceramic pot from the Chimú culture of Peru, dating to AD 1200, has also been unearthed, which shows an owl-faced woman holding a cactus. In Peru the owl is a tutelary spirit and the guardian of herbalists so the woman depicted is almost certainly a *curandera* (healer) and huachumera.

According to Ruben Orellana, a modern-day huachamero working in the Sacred Valley outside of Cusco, but also a PhD historian and one-time curator of the Machu Picchu sacred site, the first huachuma ceremonies were probably predominantly day-time affairs and, certainly at Chavín, which archaeologists now refer to as 'the birthplace of the San Pedro cult', they may well have included a sexual or tantric element since sexual and emotional arousal are other aspects of the huachuma experience and powers therefore available for magical use.

As a result of the persecutions by the Spanish, indigenous practices including the original rituals and ceremonies surrounding the use of huachuma 'undoubtedly were transformed', in the understated words of anthropologist Wade Davis.[2] In fact the use of huachuma was effectively driven underground for hundreds of years, though never completely eradicated, and those ceremonies that survived took on a new form. Firstly, the name of the medicine was changed to San Pedro – Saint Peter – 'guardian of the threshold for the Catholic Paradise...an apparent strategy of the Indians to placate the Inquisition', according to DeKorne. Secondly, the ceremonies became more secretive night-time events, which incorporated Catholic symbolism, procedures and artifacts into their rituals of healing.

I attended a number of these ceremonies in Peru in the 1990s and in my experience it is fair to say that, in contrast to the original, more joyous day-time ceremonies, the Catholic concepts of suffering to atone for our sins had also become a predominant feature of the new ritual format. Participants were first given an emetic, for example, to make them sick so they could rid themselves of 'sins' and negative energies. This was followed by a *singado* (tobacco juice snorted into the nostrils), then a bath in cold flower water, naked in the freezing night, completed by a gentle beating with *chonta* (wooden staffs) before even receiving San Pedro, which in itself was weak and insipid – and even that small gift had to be earned. Thankfully now in Peru there are curanderos who have reverted to the old ways of day-time sunlit ceremonies with strong San Pedro, which they regard as the real healer in contrast to the night-time ceremonies where the shaman and not the plant takes centre stage.

Common Reasons for Attending Ceremonies

Whether ancient or modern, by night or by day, there are fairly common reasons why someone might choose to attend a San Pedro ceremony: to cure illnesses of a spiritual, emotional, mental or physical nature, to know the future through the prophetic and divinatory qualities of the plant, to overcome sorcery or *saladera* (an inexplicable run of bad luck), to ensure success in one's ventures, to rekindle love and enthusiasm for life, and to restore one's faith or find new meaning by experiencing the world as divine. Wade Davis described a ceremony he attended in 1981, for example, where the people present included a girl who had been paralyzed, members of a family whose cattle had become diseased, a person seeking healing for a relative who had gone mad, a man who had become unstable after seeing his wife with her lover, and a businessman wanting to know who had stolen money from his company. The last reason for attending may appear to bear no similarity to the first, but in the Andean shamanic view bringing order to one's financial and business affairs and so avoiding emotional and physical dis-ease is just as valid in terms of restoring balance to the soul and peace to the mind as relieving the pains of a paralyzed girl. Both are healing in this sense. Other reasons, especially among Westerners who attend my ceremonies nowadays, are to overcome a feeling of separation, aloneness and anxiety by reconnecting with love, bliss, belonging and finding themselves at one once more with God.

San Pedro can heal all of these diseases – and sometimes instantly, with one drink alone – because, in the words of Eduardo Calderon (now deceased, but formerly one of northern Peru's most famous curanderos), it is 'in tune with...beings that have supernatural powers. Participants [in ceremonies] are set free from matter and engage in flight through cosmic regions...transported across time and distance in a rapid and safe fashion'.

He also describes the effects of the plant as this healing takes place:

First, a dreamy state...then great visions, a clearing of all the faculties...and then detachment, a type of visual force inclusive of the sixth sense, the telepathic state of transmitting oneself across time and matter, like a removal of thoughts to a distant dimension.

Thoughts arise, that's it – often deep thoughts, unencumbered by the limited rational mind, which provide answers to our diseases, dilemmas and dramas. The story behind the disease is revealed and then, in tears or in laughter, it is easy to let it go and choose a new story for ourselves, of power and wellness instead. Sounds simple – and it is, as the accounts in the next chapter show.

Healing in San Pedro (and in shamanism generally) is, incidentally, defined more widely and more usefully than Western medicine uses the term. It means an ultimately beneficial and positive change in the mental, emotional or spiritual dimensions of one's life, as well as a physical cure or change. San Pedro healing is thus more expansive and holistic, encompassing all aspects of the self, instead of dismissing the soul entirely and focusing (sometimes with disastrous results and side-effects) only on the physical *symptoms* of disease instead of its ultimate *cure*, as Western medicine does. (Again, see the next chapter for examples.)

Healing with San Pedro always takes place as part of a ceremony with the *intention* of healing – never lightly and never as a recreational 'drug experience' – and in this the *mesa* is always central.

The Mesa

The mesa (the word literally means 'table') is an altar, which may be elaborate or simple, depending on the shaman. Most are woven fabrics laid directly on the earth on which are placed power objects called *artes* ('arts') in the form of artifacts from archaeological or ritual sites to represent the ancestors, herbs and perfumes in ornate or antique bottles, which bring good luck and healing, swords and statues, stones from cemeteries and sacred places, and so on. All are meaningful to the shaman, contain energy in their own right and, more importantly, through the faith he invests in them, confer power to the shaman to do his healing work. Because mesas are personal, anything could be placed there actually. Wade Davis, in *Sacred Plants of the San Pedro Cult* lists other items he has encountered, such as wooden hardwood staffs, bones, quartz crystals, knives, toy soldiers (for the powers of opposition or victory), deer antlers and boar tusks (for strength in the face of challenges), shells, and paintings of the saints. I have also seen torches (for light), mirrors (for self-reflection or the return of evil magic) and carvings of various animals that are symbolic of particular qualities. Sometimes participants may also place an item of faith personal to them on the altar or make an offering to it.

In the traditional layout of the mesa, there are three 'fields' and where artes are placed in relation to these is significant. The left is the negative or 'extraction' field, while the right is positive and life-giving and the middle is the neutral space or 'command centre'.[3] It is important to qualify these terms, however, since negative and positive have different connotations for us in the West and may suggest a good or evil intent, which is not really present in Andean healing. Most shamans do not consider the two sides of the mesa to be good or bad, per se, for example, and, in a sense they are not even 'sides', but part of a continuum where every field is harmonious and, through their relationship to each other, ensure that the world remains in balance. Even at their extremes, the negative and positive fields complement more than oppose each other. Thus, for example, 'good' and 'bad luck' go hand-in-hand because without each we could not recognize the other.

In one way, then, the mesa can be regarded as a representation of the divine (rather than human) scales of justice where the goal is equilibrium and order and not a weighted outcome in favor of 'light' or 'dark'. This balance is important because, as shamans know, the more good luck we have (right side) the more bad luck (left side) can sometimes result as the same energy manifests in different forms, flowing from one to the other and back again. An example might be a man who has the good fortune to be wealthy and because of this indulges in fine foods and wines to the point that his desires take him over and he becomes gluttonous, ill or addicted as the energy of causality circulates. Another way of understanding the mesa, therefore, despite the linearity of its layout, is as a cosmic circle that brings everything back to its rightful place and represents the circularity of human experience.

Within this framework of understanding, the measure of a truly successful life is not riches or fine food, but a correct attitude, a moderate approach and a harmonious relationship to the physical and spiritual worlds. As if to signify this, in the centre of the mesa is the neutral field: the point of balance on which the world turns. It is also the place of transformation where illness can be cured by finding equilibrium between negative and positive forces. Herbs that bring strength and energy may be placed there, along with, for example, images of the sun (for light, brilliance and regeneration) or reflective materials and lodestones to draw in positive energies and dismiss others so that balance is restored.

Some mesas are huge, as big as a dining table and surrounded by staffs, swords and crosses; others use a different layout, are much simpler and contain fewer power objects. My own is about 12in by 12in and uses the format of a medicine wheel. My partner in San Pedro ceremonies, the Peruvian shaman La Gringa, has an even smaller mesa and her theme for the layout is evolution, moving upward from primal forces (the coiled kundalini-like serpent at the base of the spine) through the body (represented by the puma in Andean cosmology) to the condor or hummingbird, representing ascension to the higher self and the realm of angels.

Once the mesa is assembled the ceremony can begin, with the altar as the point of focus: a portal through which all energies can flow and a visual reminder to participants that the purpose of this meeting is to heal imbalances so that order prevails and the love of God can flow unimpeded. In modern ceremonies, the mesa may be 'opened' (empowered and put to work) with a simple prayer and a statement of intent. In the more traditional, Catholic-influenced ceremonies, however, the opening can be a ritual in itself.

Types of Cactus Ceremonies

According to Richard Cowan, Douglas Sharon and Kay Sharon in *Eduardo El Curandero: The Words of a Peruvian Healer*,[4] for example, Eduardo Calderón's procedure for charging and opening the mesa at the start of a ceremony involved all of the following actions.

1. *Apertura de la cuneta* ('opening of the account'). The mesa was set up in a precise way then, while invoking the forces of nature, the four winds and the four roads, Eduardo sprayed it three times with a mixture of sugar and the perfume Tabu. The same action was then repeated with sugar and the cologne agua florida, with sugar and the cologne agua kananga, and then with sugar and lime juice.

2. *Oraciones* (prayers). These were made to God, the Virgin and the saints and included the *Hail Mary* and *Our Father*.

3. *Llamada* (call). A prayer or plea was made to the *apus* (spirits of the sacred mountains) and lagoons, the ancient shrines and to curanderos alive and dead, inviting them into the ceremony. The call took the form of a *tarjo* (power

song or chant) accompanied by the shaking of a *chungana* (rattle).

4. The raising (*levantada*) of the mesa. This was done by snorting *tabaco* (tobacco macerated in aguardiente alcohol and often lime juice and honey) from a snail shell, into the nostrils, seven times for the seven 'justices' of Christ (the seven miracles in the life of Christ). Each time a short invocation was also given while, throughout the procedure, Eduardo held the Dagger of Saint Michael, the crucifix, and the rattle above his head. No tabaco could be spilled or the person doing the raising had to start again. This operation 'activated' the crucifix at the axis of Eduardo's mesa.

5. Call to the *encantos justicieros* (good charms). Eduardo sang a *tarjo* for Jesus, Mary, the apostles, saints and angels, recalling the miraculous events in their lives.

6. Raising *con las doce mil cuentas* ('with the twelve thousand accounts'). Eduardo then invoked 'the twelve thousand accounts' (powers of the mesa) and poured a shell of tabaco for each of his assistants, an operation that activated the forces for good in the positive field of the mesa.

7. *Tarjo de Jesus.* A song was sung relating to the birth, life, death and resurrection of Jesus, which was intended to invoke his presence in spirit.

8. Call and petition to God. Eduardo then raised a mixture of Holy Water and Tabu above his head and drank it before spraying the crucifix three times with Tabu.

9. Raising *con las veinticinco y doscientos cinquenta mil cuentas justicieras y ganaderas* ('with the twenty-five and two hundred fifty thousand accounts related to white and black magic').

The number 25 in curandero symbology is composed of

two 12s, each symbolizing the 11 faithful disciples plus Paul, as well as a one symbolizing Judas. Twenty-five is then multiplied by ten thousand to increase its power. In this way, Eduardo indirectly invokes the forces of evil associated with 13 to help his work (12+1=13+12=25), for these are the forces responsible for witchcraft and therefore most capable of revealing its causes. However, the forces of evil are carefully counterbalanced by the forces of good – the two 12s – in this operation, since 12+12+1 also equals 25. This raising thus activates the balanced forces of the *Centro Medio* [middle field of the mesa] and, in the process, the evil forces of the *Campo Ganadero* [negative field]. As this proceeded the assistants each snorted a shell of tabaco juice.

10. *Tarjo* addressed to the forces of nature and the ancients. Eduardo invoked the now-activated forces of both the positive and negative fields of the mesa: the mountains, lagoons, ancient shrines, streams, magical plants and curanderos alive and dead. He then sang his mesa staffs to life 'starting with the Saber of Saint Michael in the *Campo Justiciero* and ending with Satan's Bayonet in the *Campo Ganadero*'.

11. Raising the San Pedro remedy. Eduardo poured tabaco into a shell, made a cross with it over the mesa, then gave it to an assistant who bent down beside the San Pedro brew and made a cross over it with the shell before snorting the tabaco juice. This was repeated twice more, once with agua kananga and once with Tabu. The same procedure was performed by the second assistant and then the crossing and snorting of tabaco by everyone except Eduardo. If a patient could not get the tabaco into his nostrils, he could swallow it.

12. Purification and presentation of San Pedro and the

curandero to the mesa. An assistant brought a cup of San Pedro to Eduardo who placed it on the mesa in front of him. He then picked up a *seguro* (a talismanic jar of protective and healing herbs), a dagger and the cup of San Pedro and stood up. After serving themselves with one shell of tabaco each, his assistants took positions on both sides of him, and while he performed a tarjo in his own name to announce himself to God and the spirits (holding the seguro, rattle, dagger and *San Pedro* at the same time) they simultaneously moved their shells along his body from feet to waist, waist to neck, and neck to crown. Next they snorted the tabaco mixture. Eduardo then performed a *limpia* (cleansing) of himself by rubbing the seguro over his entire body from head to toes. He then sat, put everything back on the mesa and sprayed the seguro three times with agua florida, three times with Tabu and three times with kananga.

13. Yet another raising followed, this time in the name of San Pedro, performed by Eduardo with one shell of tabaco. He then lifted his cup of San Pedro from the mesa, drank it in one, massaged his head with the empty cup and blew into the cup three times. Patients then went through the same procedure of drinking their San Pedro, rubbing and blowing. Eduardo then served San Pedro to his assistants, first presenting their individual servings to the mesa and then making a benediction in the name of each one. The assistants drank, rubbing their heads and blowing into the empty cup.

14. *Limpia* (cleansing) of all present. Eduardo stood beyond the staffs of the mesa, making sure that one of his assistants occupied his seat at the mesa at all times, and the patients came before him individually so he could rub them from head to foot with the chungana,. He then blew on the rattle with a sharp expulsion of air (*sopla*). When he

had done this for everyone he performed the procedure on himself. By now it was midnight and the mesa was finally charged.

If that wasn't long-winded and distracting enough for participants, the use of the mesa in healing ('discharging the mesa') involved a further 12 stages of 'curing acts'.

1. *Purificación* (purification) of the mesa. The mesa was first sprayed with the three perfumes and sugar, the same as in the opening ceremony.

2. *Rastreo* (tracking or tracing). Then, one at a time, the patients stood in front of the mesa facing the curandero who sang a tarjo in their name while concentrating on the staffs to see which one vibrated. This staff was then given to the patient to hold in his left hand over his chest while Eduardo chanted a tarjo in the name of the staff, which was intended to activate the patient's spirit, reveal the illness and invoke the spirits that were antagonizing the patient. The song was followed by reflective silence for five or ten minutes.

3. *Cuenta* (account). Eduardo 'gazed' the patient until he was able to 'see' and then relate the events of the patient's life, interspersing his narration with questions and comments. Through this Eduardo was able to recognize and understand the causes of *dano* (witchcraft), *enredo* (love magic) or *mal suerte* (bad luck) that were bothering the patient.

4. *Desmarco* or *descuenta* ('removal or discount'). Eduardo sang a song relating to the powers of the staff.

5. Raising the patient. During the last song Eduardo's assistants had taken positions on either side of the patient and now 'raised' him from feet to waist, waist to neck, and neck to the top of the head with a shell filled with

whatever healing substance was needed to remove the cause of the patient's illness by 'centering' him.

6. Raising the staff. The patient held the staff over his head by its tip as he snorted whatever substance was specified by Eduardo. In severe cases of daño, the patient might have difficulty getting the substance down and might vomit, in which case Eduardo or one of his assistants would have to take it instead in the name of the patient. Following this Eduardo might have to perform a symbolic sword battle and perform seven somersaults (*siete mortales*) in order to defeat the witchcraft affecting the patient.

7. Cleansing the patient. Once the patient had raised the staff an assistant took it and rubbed it over the patient's body.

8. *Sopla* (blowing) and *chicotea* (violent shake) of the staff. The patient's staff was sprayed three times with whatever liquid was indicated and then used to slice the air in whatever directions the spirits suggested, before it was returned to its position at the front of the *mesa*.

9. *Salto sobre el fuego* ('leap over the fire'). Any victims of witchcraft present then had to leap four times so that their movements formed a cross over a small bonfire of straw. After the jumps they then stamped out the fire. Then, as they stepped backwards, an assistant cut the ground between his feet with one of the mesa swords. 'This appears to be a symbolic act indicating 'mastery over fire' or 'magical heat'…in order to purge and purify him or her by exorcising evil spirits.'

10. *Florecimiento* ('flowering'). For patients whose cures were nearly complete, Eduardo might conduct a final centering ritual which involved placing the patient in a circle of white cornmeal drawn on the ground, spraying holy water around the patient at the four cardinal points while

cutting the spray with a sword, and then cutting a final spray in the form of a spiral in front of the patient. After this the curandero often gave the patient advice or instructions for further healing.

11. *Cierre de la cuenta* ('closing of the account'). This is the same as the opening ceremony and was performed after Eduardo had repeated steps 1 through 8 for every person present and conducted the florecimiento and the fire ceremony reserved for victims of witchcraft.

12. *Refresco* (purification or 'refreshment'). The assistant sprayed a mixture of Holy Water, white cornmeal, white flowers, white sugar, sweet-lime juice and powdered lime in the faces, on the necks (front and back), and over the hands (front and back) of everyone, including Eduardo and each other. While they were refreshing the patients Eduardo gathered up his artes in the same order as he put them down at the beginning since all must be put away before sunrise to prevent sunlight from touching them. Any remaining San Pedro was buried for the same reason. Once it was all packed away, the curandero used his dagger to cut a cross three times in the earth where the mesa was laid, and then sprinkled the refresco mixture used by his assistants three times along the cuts and once in each of the four corners of the mesa area, which could not be touched by anyone until noon that day. All participants were required to abstain from condiments (especially salt, hot peppers, onions and garlic), pork, beans, or any plant that grows on a vine or has twisting roots until noon that day.

Having experienced some of these ceremonies (including with Julia Calderon, Eduardo's daughter, who performed a ritual similar to but different in parts from that above) I can vouch for their tedium.

While I appreciate them as a healing spectacle and for the hard work of the curandero, my criticisms are that the San Pedro given is almost always weak since the medicine is administered not as a force in its own right, but as a medium of communication between the shaman and patient, the San Pedro inside both of them acting as a channel of connection for the curandero and not the medicine to carry out the healing.

Furthermore, even if the medicine is strong, the patient is given no time to commune with it, learn from it, process the information received and begin her own healing because of the requirements of the ceremony that she attend the mesa, take part in various healing maneuvers, and then play witness to the healing of others in front of the mesa. In fact, then, these are not true *plant spirit* ceremonies, but ritualized healing procedures with the shaman at the forefront and San Pedro as one small part of the show.

During daylight ceremonies – the modern renaissance of more ancient rituals – by contrast, the mesa – simpler and more compact – is called upon, but not relied upon and may be opened and charged simply by prayer. The shaman is in service of San Pedro (which is stronger, cooked longer and charged with *fuerza*: force) instead of the other way around. Patients are given their San Pedro at the start of the event and left undisturbed to learn from and heal with the teacher plant, with the shaman intervening only when necessary or when the patient asks for help to remove a blockage they are struggling with or interpret a message from the plant. A short gathering at the end of the day serves to close the ceremony.

To each their own when it comes to choice of shaman and ceremony, but it will probably come as no surprise that I prefer the latter and this is how I conduct my own healings.

What's in the Brew?

Scientist: Mescaline.
Shaman: God.

It's as simple as that: it depends on your perspective. If you subscribe to a linear, reductionist materialistic worldview you will argue that the work of San Pedro is accomplished only by mescaline, which the cactus contains at around the one to three percent level.[5] It is this and this only that causes its effects. If you are a shaman or a ceremonial participant your experience will be that there is more to San Pedro than that and that imagining that one 'active ingredient' sums up the whole of the plant is little more than ridiculous.

In my view, it is of next-to-no value and does not aid our understanding at all to equate a plant in its totality with a summary of its constituent parts (or to single out just one) and then extrapolate from these in an attempt to explain its effects. Something gets lost when we do that, which is the 'spirit' or 'personality' of the plant. By the same token, the lifetime and actions of a man cannot be described or explained just by reference to the chemicals in his blood, the size of his brain or the lumps on his head, as other scientists and phrenologists attempted to do a few centuries ago. Besides which, experiments with pure mescaline (which were typically carried out in a sterile, clinical lab, administered by an injection to human guinea pigs by white-coated technicians with no 'spiritual' or healing context) do not produce the same results as a San Pedro ceremony. For one thing, the ceremony is missing, for another there is no shaman to guide the journey and point you towards a connection with God (or, at least, something more than yourself), for another, the intention to heal is absent, and, finally, mescaline alone just doesn't cut it.

The Scientific View

Heinrich Klüver was one of the first to study the effects of mescaline. In his *Mescal and Mechanisms of Hallucinations* (1928 and 1966) he suggested that the visual phenomena that occur under the influence of the drug are explainable simply by the structure of the brain and eye. He organized the images reported during mescaline experiments into four groups he called 'form constants': (1) tunnels and funnels, (2) spirals, (3) lattices, including honeycombs and triangles, and (4) cobwebs; concluding, in effect, that mescaline 'hallucinations' are the result of seeing patterns on the retina under the influence of the drug, with the images interpreted by (and thus generated in) the brain.

In answer to this, let me just say that in ceremony I have *never once* seen any of these 'form constants' and I have *never* heard one of my participants (and there are hundreds of them) talk about them either. Those who drink San Pedro are far more concerned with life changes, illumination and the astonishing healings and spiritual impacts that they experience, not boring tunnels and funnels.

The Shamanic View

In *Miserable Miracle*, the Belgian artist and poet Henri Michaux (1899-1984) describes his own experience with mescaline and at first, once again, gets drawn into the mechanics and visuals instead of the real *experience*. 'Hundreds of lines of force combed my being,' he wrote. 'Enormous Z's are passing through me (stripes-vibrations-zig-zags?). Then, either broken S's, or what may be their halves, incomplete O's, a little like giant eggshells.' Then something happens and towards the end of his encounter; he forgets about the patterns and edges into a deeper under-standing (one which is more obvious and immediate with San Pedro), concluding that 'one is nothing but oneself' and, '[I am] a passage, a passage in time.' Perhaps it takes an artist instead of a scientist (or at least a *non*-scientist) to appreciate the cactus-like truths that mescaline *may* contain.

The last line, I think, is key to Michaux's experience and does share something in common with San Pedro. It is not the shapes or patterns that are of importance in themselves, but the information they carry and the realizations they bring, for we are all just a passage in time, a breath on the wind, vital to the world and, at the same time, a whisper or an insignificant thought, of no more – or less – value or substance than a cloud or a blade of grass.

The sensation of being bathed or bombarded with intense colors is also common with San Pedro. Once again, however, it is not the colors that are important, but the conduits they provide for new revelations about the beauty around and within us, which is present in even the most mundane of worldly forms and the realization, therefore, that our gift of life is special.

Psychedelic explorer Terence McKenna writes in one of his books that there are '*true* hallucinations' where what we receive from visions is *more real* and operates at a deeper level than the things seen (or often not seen) in our habitual way of perceiving and processing information from the world.[6] To regard one state (normal consciousness) as 'real' and our 'hallucinatory' world as unreal and without value is therefore quite wrong. For one thing, such a distinction presupposes that there actually is a separation between the two states; that one exists in reality while the other is in some way abnormal.

Shamans see no such division. They believe that the information given to us by San Pedro, by other teacher plants or in non-ordinary states such as dreams and meditations is as valid (or more so) than that received from ordinary perception and thought. Furthermore, such information is given to us to be *used* in daily life not to be ignored, denied, or seen as lacking in merit or purpose. To deny our dreams, after all, is to deny a large part of our human and spiritual experience.

Thus, for San Pedro shamans, the visions and insights gained from the plant are there to inform our everyday behavior in the 'real world' so we can make changes, heal, or do what is necessary to improve and enhance our lives. The changes we make as a consequence of our visions mean that we become new people, closer to our real essence as 'true human beings'. This is natural and inevitable and to be welcomed as an enrichment of our condition and part of our evolution.

Archaeological and anthropological evidence points to the same unified view of life and healing on the part of ancient curanderos and huachumeros and their perception of reality as a combination of the material and immaterial, so that one informs the other. The anthropologist Peter Furst writes, for example, that the shamanic worldview does not include the notion of duality or opposing forces which split the world into two: the sacred and profane, good and bad, right and wrong. Instead, there is no purely physical world and no absolute and self-contained other-world that is wholly of the spirit. On the contrary, the curandero, in his healing rituals, seeks to find unity and balance in the inter-actions between *all* the forces of the world through a vision that can inform – and transform – his patient's life, leading to an improvement in his existence.

This view of the world is flexible enough to incorporate even seemingly-competing or contradictory elements so that a person might find as a result of his San Pedro visions, for example, that he is right *and* wrong, good *and* bad, blessed *and* cursed all at the same time. A new and expanded understanding of reality can then become part of his life through his acceptance of this unity, and his behavior (and the results that stem from it) can change as a result of the information San Pedro has given him.

In *The Doors of Perception* Aldous Huxley ruminates on the possible impact of this more unified way of seeing the world, of bringing our ordinary and non-ordinary realities together[7] when he writes that:

If we could...swallow something that would, for five or six hours each day, abolish our solitude as individuals, atone us with our fellows in a glowing exaltation of affection, and make life in all its aspects seem not only worth living, but divinely beautiful and significant, and if this heavenly, world-transfiguring drug were of such a kind that we could wake up next morning with a clear head and an undamaged constitution – then, it seems to me, all our problems (and not merely the one small problem of discovering a novel pleasure) would be wholly solved and earth would become a paradise.

True Hallucinations

There is another sense, too, in which the visionary world interconnects and co-exists with the physical world: that they are – absolutely and literally – no different from each other; that our visions are real in themselves and we do not even need, necessarily, to act upon them or *make* them real in our lives because they have a will, a vector and a volition of their own.

'Visions' and 'reality' do not just *influence* each other, that is, there are occasions when they *are* each other to the extent that a prayer, a yearning or the receipt of a blessing can itself change the nature of physical reality.

The experience of one ceremonial participant, Doris, is an example of this. Her daughter was diagnosed with polycystic ovaries when she was 13 and the doctors told she might find it impossible to conceive. In ceremony Doris asked the medicine if her daughter, now in her 20s and in a steady relationship, would ever become a mother. Doris said:

I had the clearest vision, like watching a film, of me and her boyfriend in a delivery room and her giving birth to my grandchild. I came from that vision crying with joy. My experience with San Pedro [was] the most powerful, profound experience of my life. I had *intellectually* understood about us coming from – and one day returning to – energy; I had even glimpsed this with ayahuasca, but with San Pedro I *became* energy. I completely dissolved [with] no room for ego, and breathed with the sky. I became the breath of life and infinite and eternal love and I just knew that everything would work out for my daughter and for me as well. Two weeks later, after I got home to England, I received a call from my daughter, in shock because she had just found out she was pregnant, even though she was on the pill and apparently had fertility issues! I had the vision and knew all this before she even discovered her pregnancy.

How do we explain this if San Pedro is nothing more than 'funnels and tunnels' and biochemical processes – a pregnancy that was seen first in a vision and then became true even though a medical condition and contraception made it impossible? Coincidence? The odds against it must be small. The contraceptive pill is itself 98 percent effective against pregnancy and that is without polycystic ovaries. Telepathy then? Did Doris somehow tune in to her daughter's awareness of her own pregnancy? This explanation doesn't really work either since her daughter didn't even know she was pregnant when Doris had her vision of it. Another possible explanation (although one which is now way outside the remit of science) is that the pregnancy resulted from Doris's prayers or wishful thinking amplified by the power of San Pedro.

That would seem bizarre except that Doris was not the only one of my participants who manifested her dreams in ceremony. Ben wanted to set up a charity to help people in the developing nations and needed £4,000 (about $8,000) immediately to fund a part of it. It was money he didn't have and while he was in ceremonies with me for two weeks he had left his solicitor in charge of selling his London apartment so he could raise the capital. Before our first plant ceremony, Ben set an intention for his apartment to sell so the money he needed would flow effort-lessly to him. In fact, however, when he emailed his solicitor a few days later he found that it hadn't sold at all. She did mention in passing though that, seemingly quite by chance, she had discovered a mysterious sum of money in Ben's account that neither of them knew was there. It was exactly £4,000; precisely the amount he needed. Looking at the date and time of her email and allowing for the time difference between London and Peru, where our ceremonies took place, it also turned that this myste-rious money had appeared in his account exactly at the time of the ceremony.

Reflecting on these events I am reminded of the words of Miguel, another San Pedro ceremonial guide who I met in Cusco some years ago: 'Paradise is in the plant. But we do not use San Pedro to escape there and turn our backs on this world. Instead, by absorbing its spirit, we *make* Paradise on Earth.'

But What's *In* the Brew? Meaning: How Do I Make It?

Every shaman has their own method and recipe, containing secret ingredients they never reveal to anyone. In fact, as Ruben Orellano remarks, 'The cactus itself [i.e. the spirit of San Pedro] teaches you how to make the brew, and it teaches everyone differently.' The medicine that results says more about the shaman's dedication, connection to the plant, prayers that have been made over it and good intentions put into it than any chemical process that takes place in the cooking pot.

La Gringa, a Cusco-based huachumera, explains her procedure like this:

Ruben [Orellana, her teacher] taught me a very complicated way to prepare it, but we have changed things in time. He peels and cuts the cactus then boils it for eight hours, which is how most shamans do it, but then he adds alcohol and sometimes other ingredients too. At first I thought it was very strong – and for me, of course, it was. But then San Pedro taught me another way so now I cook it for 20 hours and it is much stronger than Ruben's. Cooking it longer also means that people are much less likely to vomit when they drink it.

Other San Pedro feels weak to me now and rarely gives the same visions. Ruben says you don't really need visions for the healing to take place and he has a point, of course. But I still think they are important because as well as receiving a healing, people need to *know* they *are* healed. When the visions come they can feel it, then they understand it is real and they pay attention to what they are shown...about how to protect themselves and stay well, or their place in the world and the beauty of their lives. Without the visions they can't know this.

There are some other things to consider when preparing San Pedro as well. I usually only work with cactuses that have seven or nine spines because they produce the most gentle and beautiful brews. Those with six or eight spines are not so strong, while 11s and 13s can be very intense, but also sometimes dark. I never use either with groups. Those with four spines we only ever use for exorcisms and the patient and healer must both drink. You don't ever want to try a San Pedro like this. It is horrible and the visions take you to Hell.

While the cactus is cooking we often sing songs to it or offer our prayers that it will produce good healings. Every time we stir it we offer a new prayer, so maybe 20 prayers go into each bottle. It should never boil and the temperature must stay constant, so it is a lot of hard work.

Sometimes the spirit of San Pedro shows up while we are cooking it too, in patterns on the surface of the water which tell us who will be coming to drink it and why. I have seen patterns in the form of ovaries, for example, complete in every detail; or hearts enclosed by circles. Then the next day a woman has arrived for help with a 'fertility problem' and brought with her a man whose heart was closed to her dreams of a child. In this way San Pedro can show us what people need before they even arrive.

As we do the cooking, we are completely *in* San Pedro as well, for all of those twenty hours; so it infuses our dreams and becomes a part of us too, and we often dream of the people who will be coming to us for healing.

There are examples of various preparation and cooking methods at erowid.org8 but these are the basic steps:

1. A length of cactus measuring fingertips to elbow and as wide as your forearm makes a reasonable dose.
2. Cut this into 3in-4in chunks.
3. Cut out any spines and spine nodes then peel off the thin, plastic-like outer skin.
4. Cut towards the inner core, following the line of the ribs so you collect chunks of cactus. This means that some of the pulp will still remain, surrounding the cylindrical core. Some recipes also use this in the brew, but this part does contain a small quantity of strychnine, not enough to cause lasting damage, but enough to give you a stomach pain and irritation sometimes, so the choice is yours. This pulp makes a good shampoo though and the inner core, hollowed out and dried in the sun, can sometimes be used to make a candle holder.
5. Put the saved chunks into a pot and cover them with cold water then apply a very low heat, barely a simmer. This is also the time to add the 'secret ingredients' according to the shaman's personal recipe and to make prayers for a medicine that will answer your needs. I'm not going to reveal any secret recipes here, but I'll tell you this: tobacco adds power to all plant medicines, lime brings clarity and enables lucid dreams, and pisco (Peruvian brandy) can add potency. But, in fact, there are a million

healing plants which could be added at this point, according to your needs or desires.[9]

6. Simmer the brew for several hours, being vigilant, respectful and making your prayers throughout. The weaker San Pedros used in the night-time mesa ceremonies discussed earlier are typically brewed for around four to eight hours while those prepared for day-time use (certainly by the shamans I work with) are brewed for 20 hours or more, which adds hugely to their power.

7. Strain the mixture through gauze when it has attained a thick, mucus-like consistency and allow it to cool.

8. Drink the same day or certainly within a few days as fresh San Pedro does not keep well, even when refrigerated.

Before You Drink

All teacher plants require some ritual and sometimes medical precautions prior to and at the time of their use. This is known as *the diet* and refers not just to restrictions around food and drink, as the name might suggest, but to a prohibition on sexual and other behaviors as well, so we approach the plant with a pure intent and attitude.

Unlike ayahuasca, which may, depending on the shaman in charge of the ceremony, demand preparation some days before drinking it, as well as food and behavioral taboos, sexual absti-nence, fasting and meditation, San Pedro does not expect major changes to a participant's lifestyle. In this sense it is generally considered by shamans to be more accommodating. Nevertheless, there is a diet to be followed.

For 24 hours before San Pedro is drunk, food and drink should be as bland as possible and should not contain alcohol, meat of any kind (including chicken or fish), oils or fats, spices, citrus fruits or juices, and there should be no sex. For about 12 hours prior to the ritual, there should be no food at all. This means a day of fasting if the participant is attending a night-time ritual, or no food on the night prior to a ceremony if it is to take place the following day. For a few hours before the ritual most shamans recommend a period of quiet reflection and meditation so the participant can decide what he wants from the experience; what he would like to heal or learn about himself. Having an *intention* – a purpose for the ceremony, a healing to complete or a question to be answered – is central to all work with teacher plants and San Pedro is no exception. These are plant *doctors* and *teachers*; a ceremony is purposeful, *not* a recreational drug-taking event.

During the ceremony itself, most shamans forbid the consumption of any food or drinks apart from the medicines they prescribe. Some do, however, allow water and compatible food to be taken to the ritual (such as non-acidic fruits like banana, mango, papaya and apple, or savory, rather than sweet, biscuits). In general it is expected that participants will not eat either before or during their San Pedro experience, but some shamans accept that hunger can arise and it is better to deal with it so it does not distract from the participant's spiritual journey.

Because of the 'active ingredients' of San Pedro some health precautions are also recommended. Sympathomimetics in the cactus can raise blood pressure, for example, and other compounds may also be present which act as mild MAOIs (monoamine oxidase inhibitors) and affect serotonin levels.[10] There are also specific conditions where consultation with a shaman and medical doctor is recommended in advance of attending a San Pedro ceremony. These include problems with the colon, high blood pressure/hypertension, heart conditions, sugar diabetes and the diagnosis of a mental illness. None of these necessarily preclude the patient from taking part in a ceremony since the condition itself may be the very thing he is there to cure and, as Davis points out in his description of the ceremony performed in 1981, participants sometimes exhibit some of these very ailments, including mental and emotional imbalance. The shaman, as a healer, will, however, wish to know the problems the patient is facing.

Medical consultation is also recommended for people who are taking serotonin selective re-uptake inhibitors (SSRIs) in the form of antidepressants or drugs affecting serotonin levels as these do not combine well with MAOIs. Non-prescription medicines, such as antihistamines, dietary aids, amphetamines and their derivatives and some herbal remedies (especially those containing ephedrine, high levels of caffeine or other stimulants) should be discontinued prior to working with San Pedro.

Tobacco *is* allowed on the diet as shamans regard it as a plant doctor in its own right and a means of contacting the spirit world. It may also enhance the experience during ceremonies.[11]

Although San Pedro is more 'easy-going' than ayahuasca, for example, and there is no need to detox or diet for prolonged periods in advance of ceremonies, the experience is, in the view of many participants, enhanced by a process of purification beginning a week or so before the first ceremony. Foodstuffs normally avoided on a detox such as this include salt, limes and lemons (all of which the shamans believe to cut through magic), spices, excess meat (especially red meats and pork), refined sugar, wheat and processed foods in general. Other foods are generally considered fine on most shamanic detoxes and those recommended include vegetables such as broccoli, which supports the liver's detoxification enzymes; onions and garlic, which are good for sulfation, the main detox pathway for chemicals, drugs and food additives; artichokes to improve the digestion of fats; and beets to help regenerate liver cells, improve fat metabolism and eliminate heavy metals from the body.

Herbs and vitamins can also help the detox, although these should be discontinued a few days before the ceremony so the body is as pure as possible. Dandelion root increases the flow of bile and helps the body process toxins. Milk thistle is an antioxidant, assists in liver regeneration and neutralizes the effects of alcohol and fat consumption. Vitamin C is also antioxidant and helps to reduce some possible side-effects of a detox such as headache or nausea.

The general rule with plant work is: the purer the body and spirit the more powerful the experience of the medicine and its teachings, and the diet will certainly help.

The Role of the Shaman/Ceremonial Leader

The cactus is a powerful teacher [and] the healer must be compatible with it
Juan Navarro, huachamero.[12]

In modern daytime ceremonies (unlike the night-time events) it is not the job of the healer to do anything in particular, and certainly not to intervene in anyone's process or 'impose healing' on any participant without their request. Healing is the job of San Pedro.

Instead, the job of the shaman is more complicated and subtle since he cannot refer to a manual or a specific ritual procedure, but must relate to all ceremonial participants as *individuals* undergoing a *unique and personal* experience, and assist them accordingly. The shaman regards himself as the embodiment of San Pedro, the ambassador and representative of the spirit in the plant. He is, in effect, the human face of San Pedro; what the cactus spirit would be if it took human form. His role then is to represent and act out the qualities of the plant with a strong, quiet, dignified presence; to hold the space for participants in which San Pedro can work and to radiate a calm, assured, beneficial energy. The spiritual qualities of San Pedro might be described as strong, gentle, fearless and honest, and this is what the shaman must also be.

If healing is requested or required the shaman provides it, of course, but he does not immediately reach for the clichéd tick-box tools so overused in Western 'core shamanism' or, indeed, in more traditional Andean ceremonies, such as drums, rattles and feathers. Of course these *might* be used, as might chonta staffs, crystals and artes, but they are not automatic go-to items. Instead, the shaman relates honestly and purely to the person in front of him rather than seeing her as a 'patient' (a label) to be 'cured' (fixed by the shaman's amazing supernatural powers), so he provides whatever the patient needs in that moment. This might be counseling, herbal tea, a hug, a few words of comfort or, indeed, just sitting quietly with the participant as a witness to their courage and breakthroughs. The healing, then, is driven by the patient, not imposed on her by the shaman 'who knows best', and is therefore more empowering for the participant since she is active in her own cure and must ask for (or intimate) whatever assistance she needs to provide her own cure.

Knowing how to relate without 'technique' to each unique individual in your care, what to do and say, and how to know the spirit and intentions of San Pedro to assist the healing of the plant are skills acquired by drinking the cactus over many years and forming a bond with it, and sometimes by dieting other plants as well – like tobacco and lime – that San Pedro has an affinity with. The development of these skills requires patience and cannot be rushed.

For this reason I would not recommend that anyone reads this book and thinks they can then hold a ceremony of their own as a guide for other people. Believing so is a function of the ego, which is not compatible with San Pedro or healing work in general. Instead, concentrate on building a strong core in yourself through your own work with San Pedro and if you discover that you are truly drawn to ceremonial work, find a shaman you can apprentice with.

Chapter 2

Healing With San Pedro

'Yes, Yes, Yes, You Are Going to be Cured'[13]

San Pedro will never deceive you and he will never lie to you
Dr Valentin Hampejs, curandero

Most of us deceive ourselves. We do not live lives, but stories. If I asked you to tell me about yourself and your life over the past 40 years for example and you answered me fully and objectively then logically we would be sat together for another 40 years as you told me, moment-by-moment, all that had happened to you. This still wouldn't tell me who *you* are, of course, but I would know the events of your life and could then form my own picture of you. Even then, this picture would probably differ from your own, so maybe there is no 'you' at all in a truly objective sense?

The fact, though, of course, is that no-one does that. Nobody sits for 40 years recalling their lives in detail when they are asked about themselves. Instead, we cherry-pick moments to build a story of who we are. If we are inclined towards a 'victim' mentality, for example, we will completely overlook the ten million moments of glory in our lives in favor of another sad story; if we are narcissists we will have already forgotten our 'failures' (which will be the fault of others anyway) and the story we tell will be nothing but achievement and splendor. There is no objectivity in our summaries and synopses.

On top of this, our memories are fallible and what we choose to tell others may not even have happened at all, or not in the way we recall it. Psychologists like Elizabeth Loftus, for example, have completed studies that show that even the memories of eyewitnesses to dramatic and memorable events such as robberies and muggings are wrong in more than 50 percent of cases when they describe the event to police, recalling short, dark-haired Latino muggers as 6ft Swedish blondes, and so on. The way a question is asked also provokes a different memory response. In one experiment Loftus showed people a film of a car hitting a tree and then asked one group: 'How fast was the car going when it *smashed into* the tree?' She then asked another group: 'How fast was the car going when it *collided with* the tree?' Both had seen the same film, but the first group recalled the car travelling many miles per hour faster. She then asked both groups what color the car was. Even within the same group some said red, some blue, some couldn't remember at all. Her conclusion was that 'memory' is not a thing that actually exists, but a fluid engagement with the world through which we make sense of events. In other words, a story.

Dennis McKenna (Terence's brother) makes a similar point in his book *The Brotherhood of the Screaming Abyss*, commenting that: 'Among the most curious of my earliest remembrances are those that may not be real.' He goes on to describe an event from his early childhood where his older brother pushed him down a flight of stairs. He says:

> It's certainly a traumatic memory, but did it really happen? I have no idea. Maybe it happened to someone else and I falsely remembered the experience as mine. Or perhaps I dreamt it… I continue to be astonished by how readily the mind confabulates, creating its own story to fill in the holes in memory, to the point where I can imagine looking back at the end of life and wondering if any of it really happened.

This is how most people arrive for healing at a San Pedro ceremony: stuck in a story of themselves which may or (probably) may not actually be true and which they are (literally) sick and tired of, but don't know how to release themselves from.

They carry with them a myth of illness as part of their story of who they are. Even if they do not consciously know it, they are searching for those 'ten million moments of glory' in their lives so they can find a new story, reinvent themselves and walk out of the ritual as new people, reinvigorated and positive and ready to dream a new life instead of the same old, same old, same old...

San Pedro makes it possible for them to do so by enabling them to see through the old illusions and unstick themselves from their attachments to them so that new and more creative and healing ideas emerge.

In essence, if we are not 'real' and neither are our memories, then those parts of us that have become central to our stories and myths, but which do not serve us (for example, a belief that we are not worthy, not good enough, sick, damaged or that 'good things never happen to me'), are equally false. They are illusions we have chosen on some level to live by, but which we can now let go of in the knowledge that they also have no real meaning. Indeed, they may never have happened at all.

San Pedro shows us our stories and beyond this, that we are actually filled with a power, potential and potency, which is far greater than the lies we are telling ourselves or have been told. We can do or be anything, in fact, because we are gods and nothing is impossible for a god.

Being a God

In scientific terms, creation began with the 'Big Bang' when, from a point of singularity there was an explosion of energy into the universe, an energy that condensed into matter and created all things: the stars, the planets, the oceans, the forests, animals, plants...and *you*. We are all the same energy and all connected, one to another and to our source. What shall we call this energy, which is omnipotent, omnipresent, eternal, and from which all things came and will return? Some call it God and, for want of a better word, we may as well call it that too. And *we are that.*

In theological terms, many religions talk about a time of darkness before the beginning of the world. Then God awakens: 'Let there be light!' With this gesture polarity is created because for God to know him/her/itself there must be opposites for a measurement of being and progress to be made. According to the Bible, God then spends the next six days creating the kingdoms of the Earth: plants, animals...and *you*. Why? Because for God to learn more about what it is to be a God he/she/it requires new experiences (as do we in order to grow and know ourselves), a billion eyes, ears and senses, a billion new adventures, a billion aspects of God, one of which is you, all feeding back information on what it is to take form as a God.

Either way you look at this, then – scientifically or theologically – you're God – not even a 'child of God', but a living part of him/her/it; a fragment of the whole.

Our healing, then, is not just for ourselves, although this coming-into-power is important in its own right. Through our well-being and new understanding we become different people and we act differently in the world, touching the lives of others in new and more positive ways. Through us, ever-so-slightly, but ever-so-surely, the world changes as this new perspective ripples outwards. So this is how we really 'save the planet': not through prayer meetings or campaigns or pleading with politicians or looking for saviors, but by engaging with our own true power, changing the world for ourselves by who we are and the actions we take. By doing *something* instead of whining about *everything*. Finally, as San Pedro reminds us, we are mortal and will all be gone one day (just 'a passage in time') – which is also a reminder to make the most of what we have and get living now instead of wallowing in self-pity and despair so that we die by default each day. At the moment of our deaths some part of us will then return to God (the pool of energy that made and suffuses the universe: the architect of the 'big bang'). That God/energy will receive us and, through our experiences and the new information we carry,

God will learn more, grow wiser and evolve. Our healing, then, is not a trivial matter. Looked at in this way, the entire universe and the whole of evolution depends on it. This is the responsibility we really have as Gods. Every one of us.

Once we become aware of these things through what San Pedro does to our minds and souls, holding on to our old self-limiting stories and denying the divine in us seems ridiculous, a slap in the face to God and the behavior of children, not responsible adults with a life to get on with, things to do and enjoy and other people to serve instead of continuing with our own small tedious dramas. We become aware of our responsibilities to ourselves, each other and our planet and the need for us to grow up, to own our lives, and to reclaim the power within us which gives us the ability to do so.

San Pedro once told me in ceremony: 'I want all my children to be strong. Strong Men and Strong Women.' Not babes lost in the world but grown-ups able and willing to create and shape the world for the good of themselves and all. San Pedro teaches us (in words used in a different context by the psychologist Carl Jung) that: 'I am not *what happened to me*, I am *what I choose to become*.'

Opening the Doors of Perception

We can put all of this in a different, less 'spiritual' and more psychological way if you prefer, but the point is the same. In the words of the psychologist Dr David Luke:

When the English novelist Aldous Huxley was given mescaline (seemingly the most important psychoactive constituent of San Pedro cactus) by the English physician Dr Humphrey Osmond in 1953, he said that it allowed man access to mystical states by overriding the brain's 'reducing valve'. Huxley was a proponent of the ideas of the French philosopher Henri Bergson, who had, in the previous century, supposed that the brain acted as a filter of memory and sensory experience so that our conscious awareness wasn't overwhelmed with a mass of largely useless information, irrelevant to the survival of the organism.

Bergson suggested that if these filters were bypassed man would be capable of remembering everything he had ever experienced [i.e. of seeing his true self instead of his stories] and capable of perceiving *everything* that is happening *everywhere* in the universe [i.e. of knowing his oneness with God/universal energy]. Huxley then applied this theory to mescaline and other similar substances – which he and Osmond called 'psychedelic', meaning 'mind manifesting' – and suggested that they override the reducing valve of the brain, bypassing the filters that stop us from potentially perceiving everything. Huxley paraphrased this notion by quoting the English poet and mystic, William Blake, 'If the doors of perception were cleansed, everything would appear to man as it is, infinite.'

Simply put, to help us survive in the day-to-day world – to safely cross the road, to negotiate our relationships, to avoid conflict situations and so on – the brain filters and gates our full experience of the world (where we know and are a part of everything) because, well, immersion in the bliss-state of being one with all-that-is is not very useful when trying to avoid an oncoming bus. In the safe space of ceremony, however, San Pedro opens for us the gateways of the mind, overcoming the limitations of brain, our survival needs and our habitual selves to give us full access to the infinite wisdom we download, but ignore, every day. In this state of expanded consciousness, everything is available, everything is known, everything can be healed and everything is permitted. How we use this knowledge and power is then up to us as responsible grown-up human beings.

Healing Stories: The Accounts of Those We Have Worked With

So this, in a nutshell, is how San Pedro heals: by showing us, and allowing us to experience, *who we truly are*. The accounts below, in their own words, from those who have been healed by San Pedro, explore these truths in unique and different ways.

Changed for the better and for good

It's a complex thing to write about one's experiences with plant medicines, as each individual's experiences vary – from one person to the next, from each journey to the next, and often from each moment to the next. All I can share is my own personal experiences. However, I'm well aware that the kind of journeys I have experienced may not be the case for many. One thing of which I am certain, however, the effects of this medicine are profound and far-reaching...so profound in fact that it assures that my life, and my perspective on it, will never be the same again.

I began to journey with San Pedro at what could be considered the source, or very close to it, in the safe haven and sacred garden of the Mountain House on a mountaintop overlooking the Andean city of Cusco, under the watchful eye of huachumera La Gringa and her sons Simon and Mark, in space held by the supportive presence of the Qero paqo[14] brothers, Juan and Luis Quispe.

In the Andes of Peru, the huachuma cactus as it is known by its Quechua name, is both indigenous and traditionally used as a sacred and respected element of Andean culture. Its medicinal use can bring about deep insight and healing on physical and cellular levels as well as emotional and spiritual ones, so it was a great honor to begin this journey in its homeland and in the company of such powerful and knowledgeable guides.

To date, San Pedro has always been very gentle on me. However, I understand that is not always the case for others. At the time of writing, I have never had to surrender to a need to purge from this medicine, although I'm fully aware that may be yet to come in future ceremonies.

Ceremony takes place in the moloka, a thatch roofed round house, which is the spiritual centre of the garden at the Mountain House. Huachu-mama La Gringa sits in front of an altar and mesa with sacred objects and stones laid out alongside the tall bottles of medicine and glasses for each of the participants seated in circle around her. She speaks of the benefits of San Pedro and a little about its history and cultural significance and shares some advice and information about what one might expect from the process. A prayer of gratitude is offered to the plant spirit of the medicine and as we drink a talking stick is passed around the circle and each person is given an opportunity to share a little about themselves and offer words of gratitude and intention for their journey.

The medicine begins to take effect within 30 minutes or so with the first sensations of alteredness and perhaps a little dizziness and nausea. After the initial stage of adjustment passes and the medicine settles in the body and begins to take effect, I find my senses alter to what feels like a much higher frequency; powers of observation become more attuned, as awareness of the natural world around me takes on a different, heightened and more finely detailed dimension...the movement of clouds take on more activity and shape, birds and insects become more clearly noticeable in their activity and calls, each leaf and flower takes on a more intricate detail, as if you are able to notice everything with so much more clarity than normal. Perception is highly enhanced and a new appreciation and connection with the environment gives a sure-footedness and finely tuned awareness of all immediate surroundings.

As San Pedro works on opening the heart, I have found it has allowed me to fully appreciate even the smallest details in everything, to reconnect with all the elements of nature with new eyes and understanding and with a crystal clarity I'd never experienced before.

I know this medicine has been a key factor of profound and often remarkable healing of many medical conditions for many people and it's taken a while of consideration and contemplation as to how that has impacted on me. I can't pinpoint an exact defining moment or specific miraculous cure for me personally while journeying with San Pedro. However, I do know with absolute conviction that since my very first journey with this ancient and sacred healer plant I am changed for the better and for good; I am more calm, more grateful for all the blessings and lessons I have received, more at peace with myself and all around me, more open and loving and the occasional episodes of deep depression I have experienced in the past now really do seem a thing of the past.

It is said that once you allow the spirit of San Pedro into your life and your system, it stays with you for good. I believe this to be true and that it takes only to call upon this medicine when and wherever it is needed to re-live the journey and feel the far-reaching and ongoing benefits of working with this powerful healer and teacher plant.

Preventing cancer and overcoming self-limitations

My intention for the San Pedro ceremony was clear for me. I wanted heal my throat. For seven months I suffered swollen glands and a sore throat and being as a serious smoker I was concerned that it might be cancer. Antibiotics failed, oregano oil took down the glands a little, but the sore throat remained and I was constantly fighting the glands.

The day of ceremony I made my intention to the universe and when La Gringa offered her prayers [to open the ceremony] I saw her lock eyes with me as she said: 'You don't need me to heal you, you can heal yourself.'

It must have been 10 hours later [when the ceremony ended]

that I remembered her words and I was amazed at how much time had passed with San Pedro. Then I thought of my throat and realized it was 80 percent better.

Knowing that San Pedro keeps talking to you even days after a ceremony I said to San Pedro: 'I am listening, I know there is more for me to learn.' Then I remembered that the week before I had read a book which talked about the 'upper limit problem'. In short, we all have our personal thermostat of what amount of happiness, success or love we will allow ourselves to experience. I knew this, of course since I am a coach and when I work with clients this sort of subject often comes up, but I realized in this moment that I had never reflected on how this affected me personally. I hadn't checked my own thermostat in years!

Suddenly the penny dropped! I had gotten this sore throat the very day I had finished my most recent training and completed my website. I was in business and overjoyed! But because of my own upper limit setting, that same day I created a health problem to keep myself within my own unconscious boundary and limit the success I could achieve. The moment I made this connection my throat problem was gone! I love both that it healed and that San Pedro gave me this lesson.

It really is the most amazing journey. It shows you how you are intimately connected to all and how you have actively been creating your own lessons your whole existence. Rarely in life do we take time to lean into our emotions, to connect the dots. But when we do the truth is revealed. To help us the universe has provided us with this gift: a plant called San Pedro.

How to save a life and make money the easy way, through faith and San Pedro

I decided to go [from Mexico] to Peru for December 2014 to January 2015, but just before I got onto the plane I heard that one of my co-workers, Fernanda, aged 23, needed emergency heart surgery within the next four months or she would die, but that it would cost $350,000US, which neither her or her family could afford. On top of this, the Mexican peso had just had a big depression compared to the US dollar, so for us Mexicans that was a *really* big sum of money.

And yet it was a matter of life or death. I was really concerned, but I wasn't sure if I could do anything. I knew I had to help but I didn't know how. So I took my plane to Cusco and I drank San Pedro and I *literally* talked to God. I felt an immense kind of joy, an orgasmic one, during our conversation. God told me that I had to make a fundraiser for Fernanda, that this situation would also be an exceptional gift for me, and that all the joy I was feeling in that moment would remain with me during the whole process of fundraising.

I got pretty scared, I felt overwhelmed and very dizzy, but then God told me to have faith in myself. He also told me that I had free will and could say no to His proposal, and I was about to, but then He told me: 'For this cause I will put an Army of Angels at your service; many people will embrace the cause because of you and the Army of Angels who are about to come into your heart if you open it now and say YES.'

I ran to Mark [the shaman at the ceremony] and told him what had happened, and that I just *couldn't* do what San Pedro and God were asking of me and he just said: 'Well, sorry, but if san Pedro tells you to do something you MUST do it!' Then I looked up and saw an Army of Angels commanded by four big Archangels, they were dancing in the sky and flying towards me. So I said YES.

Then I began to panic at my commitment to God and I asked myself a lot of questions, like how should I start? What should I do? Because I had never raised money for any cause before. Through San Pedro, God answered me. He told me to keep my eyes and heart open and that ideas would pop into my head, amazing people would enter my life and help make it happen, and the Army of Angels would remain with me until March 20 and on that day I would have all the money Fernanda needed.

So I got back to Mexico excited, but still with no idea how to start. I told my friends Michelle, Georgina, Macarena and Rosy what had happened and invited them to help me and without blinking an eye or asking any questions they all said YES. I understood then that *they* were the four Archangels I had seen on San Pedro day, and they were leading other Angels. Yet out the four of them, only Macarena knew about fundraising.

The first days were difficult, we didn't know how to start; no one in the campaign knew how to do it. So on January 22 I went and saw Fernanda and I took a piece of paper and wrote a prayer on it: 'I want her heart to keep beating. Please help us. *Latiendo Por Fer* (Beating For Fer)' and I asked a girl from our office to take our picture with the sign. The girl was really moved so after taking our picture she said: 'I also want a picture with Fernanda and that sign to put on my Facebook page.' So that's how everything began, suddenly all the office was taking pictures with my sign and Fernanda and uploading them on their Facebook pages to help us raise money. That was the first time I saw the Army of Angels in action.

One day we got call from an important guy in Mexico who must have seen this. He promised us a big donation, but he wasn't able to meet us for days and I became so disappointed and tired after going every day to his home to try to see him. We were already in February and God had told me in the San Pedro ceremony that the Army of Angels would only remain with me until March 20 and the campaign would end then, yet we had only raised $22,929 US so far. That night I cried in anguish and I dared to tell God: 'I am out now, I'm done!' But still the next day I went again to try to see the guy, saying to myself all the time: 'This is the last time you try with this guy.' And guess what, it really was the last time because on that day he could see me and he gave me $60,000US!

But the most exciting thing of that day was still about to

happen. After giving me the donation he invited me into one of his favorite rooms. It turns out that he was an Angel collector! It was a beautiful room with figures of Angels everywhere. Archangels, Angels, cherubs, on tables, on walls, on shelves, EVERYWHERE! The experience of my San Pedro day in Peru came back to me and I just felt the same amazing joy again. It was a pretty clear message to me: 'There is an Army of Angels behind you. Do not give up!'

So a lot of Angels came into the campaign, we called them Urban Angels. There were still some very difficult days as we all felt the stress at the core of *Latiendo Por Fer* – fights, tears, dramas, etc, but every time I nearly said again: 'I am really done with this now, I am out!' God sent me help. National TV shows came knocking to interview Fernanda about her condition, newspapers got interested. One time a national paper actually used the headline 'An Army of Angels are doing everything they can to save Fernanda'. I told nobody about the Army of Angels that I saw in Cusco so it was clearly another message for me. Keep going.

Then God sent me another gift. After three really bad days we got a call from Molotov, my favorite rock band of all time! They joined the cause and began doing concerts for Fernanda and from the stage they asked their fans to buy the little heart-shaped keyrings we had had made with the slogan *Latiendo Por Fer: Beating For Fer*. As an extra gift for me I got to meet the band, my heroes, several times!

In Cusco God really told me the truth that during the campaign I would feel the same orgasmic joy that I felt at the San Pedro ceremony, without even taking any substance at all. That feeling is so amazing that I do not have words in English or in Spanish to describe it.

Then came March 20 and just as God had promised, we made it. In fact we crossed the goal and on that day we had $361,214US! Fernanda had her surgery and she is ALIVE!!!

Fernanda's last words to me before she flew to Rochester Mayo Clinic were: 'You are a superhero, thank you for saving my life,' and I felt it for real then – because I really did. Me! I saved someone's life! Her father's words to me were: 'Thank you for being a sister and mother to my child.'

Other than doctors very few people have the grace to save a human life and I am so grateful to San Pedro because it showed me how I could and it cleaned and revived my relationship with God on such a level that I could trust in His plans for me and follow His instructions. Nowadays, many of us have lost our connection to God, to our Mother Earth and even to our humanity. For me San Pedro was the KEY to open the door to where my humanity was hidden and to realize that I am an important piece in the world and that if I listen to God and the divine in myself I will be free and infinitely happy – as I am right now. San Pedro showed me that nothing is impossible.

Ana Limon

NEVER
EVER
EVER
GIVE UP

Walking again

Tomas, the author here, drank San Pedro with La Gringa at her Mountain House near the Temple of the Moon. He arrived using a walking stick and found movement difficult. At the end of the day he threw away his cane and began to walk almost normally.

To give a little introduction to 'what happened to me' and how I was before, I had surgery for a cyst inside my spinal cord at the cervical level, which left a scar on my spine that led to difficulty moving my left side and to sensory alterations, like feeling my limbs numb, or even not feeling pain, heat or cold on my right arm, legs and feet, like I was floating on a cloud. Sometimes it was hard to place my left foot on the ground without direct view of it. All this was really improved with San Pedro.

San Pedro was most healing for my nervous system. [After drinking it] I started feeling the pressure of the floor on my feet, my muscles relaxed, and I recovered a lot of sensitivity in my body. [It felt like] six months of [physio]therapy in that single week. San Pedro also helped me realize I can trust my body, and that helps a lot at moving around.

I [still] go slowly, but with better movement quality, which is what matters. I even started using my left hand in more tasks like typing in the cellphone or holding the railing of the bus when I travel standing, and I reach higher things now like cabinet doors or washing my head with my left arm, so I really got in charge of my recovery. Things have been clearing up and I know that if I could do more with San Pedro it would get me healed in no time.

Healing epilepsy and addiction by loving oneself

Back in April 2015 I was very ill, physically and mentally. I was addicted to opiate painkillers prescribed by my doctor and had been taking very large doses of Codeine every day since 2006. I was taking Clobazam and Epilim to reduce the amount of petit mal and grand mal epileptic seizures I was having. I was diagnosed with post-traumatic stress disorder (PTSD) in 2009 and had been taking 200mg of Sertraline (an SRI antidepressant) ever since my diagnosis. I was taking Calci-chew tablets every day and an Andrenoic Acid tablet every week for osteoporosis. I was taking Omeprazole capsules every day for heartburn/gastro problems. I had been using a steroid inhaler every day and I was using my blue Salbutamol several times a day. My mum had been told by a kidney specialist that she had 12 months to live and my dad, who was mum's full-time carer, had started having symptoms of dementia. I felt powerless and deeply depressed, I was just waiting for my mum and dad to die before I could give myself permission to end my own life. I have always been an introvert, but I was now so withdrawn I had almost become agoraphobic, only leaving my parent's home on a Monday to work for Amnesty International and once a month I'd travel up to Birmingham. My mum had become an agoraphobic after my nan and granddad died when I was 10 and now I was the one who found it very challenging to leave the house.

I had read a lot about an English-born shaman called Ross Heaven and the plant teachers he used with his clients – salvia, ayahuasca and San Pedro. I knew that thousands of people had experienced amazing healings with ayahuasca and San Pedro. I cashed in my savings and booked on a 10-day course, 'The Three Great Plant Teachers', with Ross in Spain. Ross sent me an information pack via email and informed me that I had stop taking my SRI anti-depressants at least a month before drinking ayahuasca and to stop taking opiates. I gradually cut down my dose of Sertraline and starting taking kratom as I slowly lowered my dose of Codeine. I took my last Sertraline tablet at the end of May, but unfortunately I was now addicted to kratom, taking larger and larger doses. I had managed to come off the opiates early, but I had simply swapped one addiction for another. As soon as the kratom started to wear off I felt very depressed and I was in a lot of back pain. By the start of July I was taking a large dose of kratom three times a day. I stopped taking kratom when I started my strict plant-based diet a week before I left for Spain.

When I woke up in Spain, I was so depressed I didn't realize how lucky I was, with the benefit of hindsight. I had my breakfast (porridge oats with water) in a gorgeous valley surrounded by beautiful mountains, trees and flowers underneath blue skies with lovely warm Spanish sunshine. I was feeling very anxious and my whole body was aching. I put on a brave face and acted confident as I met others who were on the 10-day course and finally met the shaman – Ross Heaven. I was surprised how nice and friendly he was when he shook my hand, he smiled and said: 'Hi I'm Ross.'

After following Ross on Facebook for a long time, I was expecting a more provocative and less compassionate person.

After breakfast we all had a circle meeting, Ross introduced himself and described his background from Big Pharma salesman to shaman. Then each participant introduced her or himself, going around the circle one person at a time and explaining why they were there. I was getting more and more anxious as it got closer to my turn to speak. I almost had to run to the toilet and I was thinking to myself: 'Who the F*** are you?', 'I don't belong here!' and 'I am nothing.' Stupid stories I had been telling myself for years were running through my head. As I began to introduce myself I decided to share my most shameful secret to a group of strangers, something I had never talked about before. I was sexually abused by my 'bodybuilding coach' when I was a teenager and had felt too ashamed to tell anyone for over 20 years. Once I said it, I poured it all out and felt a huge sense of relief. Everyone in the room was compassionate and non-judgmental.

On the evening of my first ayahuasca journey, Ross advised me to drink only half a cup because I was taking epilepsy medication and because of my history of having seizures. I drank half a cup of the medicine and after what seemed a very long time of hearing a lot of crying and purging in the room, the shaman asked if anyone would like a second cup. As soon as I drank my second half cup I lay back in my position in the circle in the pitch black feeling very nauseous and suffering from a stomach ache. Within a few minutes Ross starting singing a beautiful icaro next to me and my visions started. I first saw flashing lights in the distance and as they got closer I noticed they moved and looked like snakes. Up until that moment I had had a phobia of all snakes (not just the dangerous ones) and suddenly I realized how silly that was. I then felt Ross tapping my stomach with what felt like bamboo leaves while singing another beautiful icaro. Ross then did some more healing on my stomach and my stomach ache was gone. Ross held my head and my visions got a lot more intense as he sucked the side of my head and purged out my epilepsy.

I had very vivid visions of my brain and the snakes were now neurons travelling through my brain. When Ross sang the words 'choose one' from his icaro for the 'Thousands of Healing Flowers', ayahuasca showed me tobacco and that I didn't need to take any drugs for epilepsy. I had only started smoking two days before my ayahuasca journey and my rational mind had been struggling with it until that point. Ayahuasca helped me understand that smoking additive-free natural tobacco was good for me and I have smoked ever since.

I also haven't taken any medication since that day three months ago. I realized that all health problems are psychosomatic. I had created all of my health problems due to my belief system and by not dealing with old traumas. I had previously heard 'new-agers' talk of *dis-ease*. I hadn't felt at ease since I was 10 when my nan and granddad were still alive. This was also the time I had begun to feel very small and weak, which led to decades of body dysmorphia. No matter how big and strong I got, I always felt small and weak. If I loved myself, loved my body, I would finally feel at ease with myself. Things would get easier and flow better.

I came home from Spain on a real high. I was now medication/drug free for the first time in over 25 years. I was feeling very happy, healthy and optimistic. Unfortunately when I told my family that I no longer needed my medication they thought I had gone mad and started to worry about me. My sister got angry with me and a friend made fun of what he called my 'Psychedelic Detox' in Spain. He saw it as a contradiction and an 'oxymoron'. I felt frustrated that people lacked faith in my healing, but they had plenty of faith in Big Pharma and Western medicine. My frustration gradually turned to depression, insomnia and losing my confidence again. I realized I had a lot more healing work to do and paid my deposit to attend a shamanic healing retreat with Ross Heaven and La Gringa in Peru. I set part of my intention for the trip to find the strength to care for my parents while shielding myself against (what I then considered) their 'doom and gloom negativity'...

After drinking San Pedro [in Peru] though, I realized that *I* needed to change, not my parents or anybody else.

I sat on a really comfortable swing seat in the Mountain House garden with my arms stretched out to my sides while stretching out my back. I had a vision of Jesus being crucified on the cross and imagined how he must have felt. While he was being tortured/crucified, Jesus said: 'Forgive them, they don't know what they're doing.' I thought about everyone who had ever hurt me and everyone I'd hurt in my life. Every single person who had hurt me had themselves been hurt. They didn't know what they were doing. Meanwhile, I was projecting my 'shadow' and emotionally reacting when I upset others. I decided to forgive everyone, including myself. The Kingdom of God is Within *You*, within all of us. Everybody I meet is a potential teacher who has God within them. I decided to stay humble and to listen and learn from everyone I meet...

My last San Pedro journey was the most healing day of my life. As the effects began I had a memory of the last time I went to my nan and granddad's flat. It was a week before my nan died of an asthma attack and three weeks before my granddad died from bladder cancer. I was 10 years old and I remember standing next to my granddad in the bathroom, he was urinating blood, out of breath and looked in pain. I was so shocked I didn't say anything and acted as if everything was normal. I remembered my dad breaking the news of my nan's death to my mum a week later and how much I wanted to take away mum's pain. I remembered how weak and useless I felt at the time.

I still felt weak and useless when I won numerous bodybuilding contests years later. I felt like a loser and became depressed after I only placed 2nd in the Mr Britain contest. After nearly 30 years of martial arts training, 14 years of working in the security industry, on the doors in pubs and clubs, I still had a lot of fear and very little real confidence (only macho acting). I then remembered the last time I saw my granddad, he was in hospital and having a blood transfusion. I felt very shy and sad, I couldn't speak. I just sat on the ward next to my granddad's bed and stared at the TV. There was no sound and my dad said: 'Why don't you ask granddad if he can get someone to turn up the volume?' I just shook my head and carried on watching the TV, trying to distract myself from looking at my granddad. Before I left with my mum and dad I gave my granddad a kiss, but I couldn't say 'Goodbye'.

I cried uncontrollably as I remembered all of that and carried on crying for what seemed like a long time. I felt that my nan and granddad's spirit was with me in the ceremony room, I clearly visualized them both and said 'Goodbye' to them. I felt a pain in the back of my head all the time I was crying. I realized I had been stopping myself from crying since I was 10 and that was what caused me to have epilepsy. As I realized this, I had a strong smell of agua florida and opened my eyes. Ross was sat next to me and poured some into my hands. I put my hands to my face, took a deep breath in through my nose and rubbed the agua florida into the back of my head. I quietly told Ross about my headache and how I had stopped myself from crying for decades. Ross did some healing on my head, my headache disappeared and I felt a rush of pleasant light-headedness – a kind of dizziness as all the decades of stress left my head. I realized I had been shy since I was 10 and there was no need to feel shy anymore. I went into the garden to smoke and I realized what a powerful, loving, confident man I really am – a Wounded Healer.

I have made sure every person I have come into contact with since that day has gone away feeling a little bit better. I have made new friends and now enjoy meeting new people and chatting with customers at the Amnesty International shop where I volunteer. I have written a couple of short sci-fi stories, I make up songs and games for my nieces every day and I have love and respect for everyone I meet. I feel at peace with myself for the first time in my life – and this is just the beginning. 'I can see clearly now the rain has gone, I see all obstacles in my way...' San Pedro taught me how to do that and the great Grandfather is flowing through me every day.

My dad's dementia and mum's illness are a still bit of a challenge for me, although I haven't felt angry or depressed once since getting home. I am looking forward to my 40th birthday next year and I'm very optimistic about my future. Thank you Ross, thank you La Gringa and most of all thank you Granddad Pedro. I thought ayahuasca was magic, but San Pedro is the ultimate healer.

Life got more worth living

I was blessed with a healing from San Pedro that I did not expect and my life is so much better for it. I have suffered from acid reflux for over 10 years and ever since the San Pedro ceremony I have been free, cured of it. I used to be nervous to eat just about everything because it meant much discomfort and pain, but now I can basically eat and drink anything and this is now over five months later. I can eat without fear. And I have been!

There are no failures or mistakes

I have been very blessed in my life with the opportunity to experience many adventures and having many great people cross my path. I have stood on Everest and sat under the Bodhi tree. I spent months in Buddhist monasteries high in the Himalayas and have jumped out of planes. Moreover, I have been lucky enough to obtain a decent amount of 'success' as it is defined by our culture. Even more importantly, I have been blessed with a wonderful partner and wife with whom I get to enjoy the greatest gifts of my life – in our two kids. So on the surface everything looked great. Yet, despite the outward appearance, all was not well deep down inside my being.

There were holes as I call them. These holes were created by events of childhood, a conditioned belief system that did not reflect how life truly worked (most of us in the 'west' have this mindset) and I also had the guilt and fear brought on by religious conditioning at a young age. These holes were a by-product of fear and pain, which was a result of incorrect thinking and ignorance. Somehow I managed to hide the fear pretty well from others and even myself at times. But it was always present. The pain caused by this incorrect thought pattern kept me in continual search for a way out of the suffering.

Of course, like so many others who suffer from this delusion, I tried finding relief through religion, philosophy, adventure, relationships, drugs, alcohol, power, money, etc. There were moments where I had what I thought were good times, but it was all transitory. In the end, not only did I make a ton of stupid mistakes, but I managed to hurt myself and others as I stumbled through this existence. Fortunately, there had been a few moments of clarity found while sitting with Buddhist monks or communing with nature and at times through the enlightened words of sages from the past and present. Yet there was never anything to help bring lasting clarity to the confused mind or peace to a tormented heart. The anger, the resentment, the confusion, the pain and the fear persisted in the centre of my being. Despite having much to be grateful for I was deeply unhappy and I held a lot of misplaced resentment. As I began to awaken to see the delusion of my thought process, I also began to see the cracks in the matrix that our culture has become. Of course, this new insight only brought more despair since it became clear to me that everything that I once thought I could count on was really just an illusion.

For those that have been to this place, you know that it is not fun. I could no longer hide from myself. Making matters worse was the fact that I had already tried all the other vehicles I was aware of to find some peace and understanding. As such I did not think there was any realistic way I could get the answers I needed to bring some relief. I was slowly dying inside while I was slowing killing myself with alcohol and anger. Anyway, you get the picture. Even though the outside looked like I had it all and all together, it wasn't pretty on the inside.

I remember one night lying in bed reflecting on all of the government corruption, on how apathetic our society has become within a culture that has gone off the deep end. Out of frustration and lack of understanding I reached a point in my life where I had to question the very fabric of existence. My resounding question to myself was: 'What is the point of it all?' To be clear, I had no plans to end my life, but I really could not get my head around why the world was so screwed up, why people behave the way they do (myself included) and why I was so miserable deep inside. There really did not seem to be any real reason to live outside of the fact that I had two kids that I had to take care of and who counted on me to guide them. But, how on earth could I possibly guide them through this mess of a life, especially when I had no real answers?

Then, as it so often happens, just when I was about to give up on finding some solutions I came across La Gringa's work. As I learned more about her and the amazing plant San Pedro, I knew I had to go to Peru. Within two months I was there at La Gringa's with her kind heart of an angel wide open to me, my wife and the other participates who gathered at her sacred garden just steps away from the energetically charged Temple of the Moon. What a special woman and a special place to ingest what would turn out to be an amazing teacher.

Grandfather San Pedro stepped into my life that stunningly beautiful day in the Andes and he has never left. The medicine showed me how all the dots in one's life connect and how we are all connected. On that day I clearly saw and spoke to my parents, both of whom had been deceased for over 10 years. Through that communication I was able to completely let go of the resentment that had been destroying me. Through this medicine I was able to understand how they (like all of us) did the best they could based on their level of understanding. I could see how everything in my life led me to that moment in time and how there was no failures or mistakes. There was no need to hold anything but love for them or anyone else for that matter. Moreover, I saw that they were not separate from me but they *were* me and I was them.

There were many powerful insights that day, all given in a very loving and gentle way. It is no wonder San Pedro is referred to as Grandfather. I never had one, but if I did I would want him to display the same characteristics of love, wisdom and compassion. That day was filled with amazing events and teachings, but one of the most poignant was coming to the under-standing that no-one and nothing can heal us. We each heal ourselves. The power is truly within. In fact, the medicine allows one to realize that there is nothing truly outside of ourselves – there is no separation, we are all of it. Additionally, I understood that we are here to learn, to grow and when we remember how amazing we truly are the struggle subsides and we can see life and our place in it much more clearly. This clarity allows one to see how all the dots connect and that it is all good (even when we think it is not). In the end I could see that we are perfect in our humanness, in our frailty and in our imperfections. It is all perfectly imperfect.

Of course, one must continue to do his/her own work as there is no magic bullet. But San Pedro is a powerful tool to help one see who they really are and to help one change perspectives so that the events of our lives become empowering instead of debilitating. For anyone who is called to this medicine I would highly encourage you to step into the unknown and discover your true self and allow San Pedro to guide you back to your own magnificence.

Unsticking yourself

In the ceremony my soul was pissed off with current path. Inner self was really angry and sad. Tears came, a message came: 'Why are you doing this job? It is causing you so much pain and is making you ill.'

Since that day I have taken months to unstick myself from my job, but I have done it! I quit at Easter. I had been a primary teacher for 11 years... Full on... Missed out on my daughter's years being 10 upwards because my energies were being ploughed into this crazy job of endless tasks and ongoing multi-tasking to make you spin... I have had to work a three-month notice as that is how it is in teaching, but ever since I have felt ill and wonderful... Noticing how ill this makes me feel has *made* me feel wonderful as I know I am now on the right path... Freeing my soul at last. (My first thoughts when I got my first teaching position wasn't happiness, but that I had sold my soul...now I am being given the chance to reclaim it!)

In ceremony my own insecurities were also mentioned – loss of James, of him running off with someone, saw in him a need to play, asked why he felt he needed to look after me, he said it was his job. An event occurred, leading my belief that perhaps James needs to learn to *receive* love. I get the rejected feeling from him, but I needed to realize *this comes from ME!* San Pedro was telling me to keep communicating, listening attentively, learn from each misunderstanding and not to go round in circles again and again.... Change something, realize *the truth*, not what you perceive it to be...

[I] said to James that I felt like I had transcended...seeing connections between trees, connecting with each other, saw our breath and how our breath affects everything around it, moves the air around, which journeys away affecting everything. I saw everything as energy. And how everything affects everything with its energy. Drums, fire, from a distance...it all dances to the music, I saw how everything is the same thing. We watched the stars dance in the sky, felt close to everything.

Messages which came a few days/weeks later were... Fill up the self with love so you can share your best energies with others, the most important things in life. Are *your people* around you? Do not give your energies to things that simply don't matter, don't mean anything...

Since quitting work and much talking to James (we have shared so much more) I am following this path with no resistance from the universe... It is just flowing beautifully. I have also apologized and acknowledged to Jasmine (my 21-year-old daughter) my sorrow and regret for putting my energies into the financial securities and not her emotional wellbeing when she was younger... But not with a guilty load. She understood, we both let it go...

I feel so brilliant about the huge life change, my huge change in how I am able to give love, knowing how full of love I am and knowing I am going to channel it to the things and ones that really matter...

Of course this is only since amazing transformations happened in Peru with my first ceremonies where I grew a new core to my being when San Pedro made me let go of a lot of shit! Wow! Thank you – how wonderful that people all over the world can share healing with this wonderful medicine... Thanks to you. And of course Mr San Pedro himself...

Rebirth into who I am

I want to tell you everything San Pedro showed me. I was a little discouraged yesterday when I randomly heard it is very important to keep your feet on the ground when drinking San Pedro – this is exactly what I enjoyed the most NOT doing! Anyhow, I believe there is no wrong way to go, the more one can open, the more one will see and experience and that can only be wonderful right?

It's difficult to put in words what I have seen and experienced with San Pedro. It's taken me so much further than words can ever say and still today I keep learning from it. My first San Pedro experience was very physical. I could feel San Pedro caressing every part, cell, of my body, it was a WOW feeling. My intention before I drank was for San Pedro to show me a way to be happy and I could not stop smiling for 12 hours. It was more than a happy feeling, it was a complete connection with everything around me, especially nature. Sometimes the love coming from the plants and trees was just overwhelming. It was a connection with my own love and the love of the universe and our planet, and it was all just beautiful. I had also put intentions into healing my past and to make me understand why I had to go through the things I have. San Pedro did show me, but it wasn't until the second time I drank San Pedro that I fully understood the answers San Pedro had given.

On my first session I was experiencing a complete rebirth, I saw myself as a new-born or before I was born, and I felt contractions and problems breathing. I was giving birth to myself, it was confusing and beautiful at the same time. I have never given birth before so I didn't know how to interpret this until days later. I believe San Pedro showed me myself in my purest state to understand who I am and that no matter what happens to me along the way I have to remember who I am. I also believe San Pedro wanted to give me a fresh start, a new beginning, a second chance and to show me I am always able to change my life whenever I want to. Also San Pedro showed me clearly that my future now is much more important to me than my past and I need to let go of my past sufferings to put that energy into *this* moment and the future. I also had almost a 12-hour orgasm, very nice! It was well needed and reminded me my body is not only a vessel and to not forget about my own pleasures and to enjoy this wonderful body given to me.

I didn't know if this was unusual or weird as my experience was nothing like my friends' experiences. It wasn't until my second San Pedro session that you told me San Pedro is rebirth. My second San Pedro experience was not so physical but more astral. I was traveling back in my past lives. I was now able to understand why I have scars on my lungs, something that has been hurting me for as long as they have appeared, at age 13. Before that I was abused by my brother so I never understood why I had to live through all these physical and mental sufferings. This time San Pedro was very clear in showing me why I had these problems breathing. I felt I was in Egypt and I saw this young girl laying in a coffin which was almost formed around her body. I was feeling proud, full of energy, confused and very afraid and panicked all at the same time. I was panicking because I couldn't breathe as I was buried alive. I could see my brother crying over my grave, devastated for losing me. That explains to me why he came back to me as my brother in this life and why he has the feelings for me that he does. All this information came to me very clearly and to me it made perfect sense. I didn't know how to comfort the girl in the coffin. I tried breathing for her, held her hand. I even told her she can come with me and be part of me and experience love in this life with me. I felt as if she was sad because she would miss out on love and to have a family so I promised her she will have all that with me in this life. I can feel her being part of me now.

The little death

I had a very profound and beautiful San Pedro connection and experience. Nothing quite prepared me for it. I am glad to have been guided through this cathartic experience and could not have done it on my own. The plant does need that respect and experience of guidance, no doubt about that.

My experience is quite difficult to put into words, but my fear of letting my heart open was intense and when I surrendered to

San Pedro my emotions were quite overwhelming to say the least. When the moment passed I felt an immense relief and deep sense of inner peace. Also waves of what I could only describe as an orgasm continued for many hours after the catharsis. During my intense emotional outburst I saw and had been seeing blood vessels which seemed to be inside my body. And these seemed to fill up with blood and white light before and during this experience. I can only think it may have been stagnant energy within my body. Who knows? But it does not matter as the body will know what to do with it.

After that I continued to feel extremely tired, exhausted, and experienced San Pedro talking to me. He told me to stay with him and that he knows everything and will heal my body. I noticed throughout the rest of the day feelings of contraction and then relaxation throughout my whole body.

I continue to experience emotions and memories returning within my body. Today I had another heart-felt emotion of intense feelings of death, like I had died, and I sobbed. It's like my heart has known death and now rebirth and that life will not be quite the same now after San Pedro!

I needed to love and take care of myself
I have struggled with severe physical and emotional 'dis-ease' most of my life. Now, after my work with San Pedro, I don't even associate with it anymore. We become so attached to our diseases (like protection or a badge of honor) and they can be hard to let go. I just needed to learn to love and take care of myself as the person I am...and now I know I don't need a disease to do that. I am SO grateful to San Pedro.

Worthy of love and belonging
I am more alive than I have ever been. I am free. I had caged myself for so many years. To feel is scary because it is my edge. For so long I have stayed safely back, bound to my own limitations

and not seeing the chains. I see them now, and they are many. Do I peel them off one by one, measuring each and feeling its weight lift? Do I explode out all at once, shattering everything in a fury of fierce freedom? Or do I glide smoothly out of them, see them slide off me like water, a clean emergence into myself?

The lines on my hands are my journey, and it has been weary at times. But I am grateful for that too, as that is where I find my strength. Where the lines cross a new layer can be formed. I let the wind fill me and take comfort in my skin. I am what I was always meant to be.

The facets of my being take pleasure in the light. I play and explore and dance with my edges. I am a continually renewing understanding of myself. The stories of my life wrap around me as I cultivate the foundation for my person. I awaken the power within me and I am humbled. It was only ever caged by fear. It is a slow and steady march, this life. A deliberate pace is needed as the world circles us in a frenzy – chaotic spokes, but we are the hub. It is effortless and it is everything I have. It is self-sustaining. It is my highest form. I am imperfect and I'm wired for struggle. But I am worthy of love and belonging.

The healing after the healing (1)

I feel such a love for San Pedro. Every single night since the ceremony I've been shown new things about myself – I'm looking forward to going to bed every night, it's like going to the school I always wanted to go to where I learn the real and interesting things! A couple of days ago I woke up and was so surprised that there was no-one in my room because I felt I had been talking to someone all night. The loving spirit of San Pedro.

The healing after the healing (2)

The journey continues, I can't explain the how or what, only that it is happening and I am seeing glimpses and moving and flowing within it. I wish I had the words of a poet to express the wonder of it all. I have none. I thought of the great masters and the paintings that have moved me, there is none that can compare. As you said there is no going back and why would you ever want to? How incredibly exquisite.

Healing Themes: What is San Pedro Here to Teach Us?

Certain motifs tend to recur in encounters with San Pedro, which in one way or another also thread their way through the healing accounts above. These are some of the core teachings of the cactus spirit.

We are all as perfect as we can be in this moment

Given all that has happened to us, the circumstances of our lives, our wounds and sorrows, 'triumphs' and 'failures', we did the best we could at the time and we should not blame ourselves or others for what we consider to be our pains and mistakes. Let go of the guilt and shame. Let go of the blame. We are human. We are all striving to give and receive love. This is the force that really motivates us and we must not lose sight of that. We are all as perfect as we can be in this moment – *and we can be more perfect still in the next.*

There is only now

There is no 'past'. It is gone and can never return. It cannot caution us or warn or inform us because those unique circumstances and events will never arise again. What we cling to is a memory – and memories are fallible, so what we are really holding on to is illusion.

There is no 'future'. We *create* the future second-by-second with every choice we make. No matter how trivial that choice seems it opens a new doorway for us and leads us onto a new path. Where that path leads we cannot know until we make the next choice in the next moment.

Now is all we have. So let go of fear, of worry, of self-limitations and *live it.*

Respect the choices you make; honor your commitments; tell the truth and take responsibility for your actions

Nobody forces us to make a commitment or a promise to others, or to ourselves for that matter. It is our choice. But when that commitment is made we must stand by it in order to build our core and our character, without which we are nothing. The truth is that we *can* have anything we want. The modern world shows us this every day in its preoccupation with instant gratification: everything is available right this second, and really there is nothing wrong with that; life is to be enjoyed.

What the world doesn't teach us, however, is how to take responsibility for what we have chosen. And so we consume everything unthinkingly, and take what we have for granted, giving it no further nourishment or attention once it ceases to interest us – including our relationships to ourselves and others and to our planet. We are grooms standing at the altar about to say 'I do' while eyeing up the bride's sister. Desire never stops, but what of the consequences when we get what we want? We act like children: we crave and act from desire, but refuse to own our actions.

We are bigger and better than that. The modern world has convinced otherwise and taught us that we are small, powerless and insignificant, that our actions don't matter so we can behave how we want. But the truth is very different. We are Gods. We *create* this world by what we think, say and do. Taking back our power and changing the prevailing mentality of the world starts with individuals taking responsibility for the consequences of their choices, as grown-ups.

Be grateful for what you have

The world has also convinced us to live in fear of scarcity and so our prayers are filled with wants and desires, our focus on being rescued – from illness, lack and loss. This, paradoxically, only strengthens our dis-eases and fuels the fear that underlies them because of all the attention we give to what we do not have. If we are looking for *real* changes in our lives and new results in the world, however, it is not just a 'spiritual practice' but common-sense to be thankful for the things we have instead of complaining about what is missing, because by placing grateful attention on these things we empower them to empower us. Like all of us, God prefers the prayers of the grateful to the whining of needy children and is more inclined to provide more of the same to those who appreciate His offerings.

And then, on another level, who are you praying to anyway when you ask for the things you don't have? Only yourself. So you may as well forego the pointless pleading and take back your power by being the answer your own prayers. In the words of George Bernard Shaw (*The True Joy of Life*) be 'a force of nature instead of a feverish, selfish little clod of ailments and griev-ances, complaining that the world will not devote itself to making you happy'.

Choose life

Dr Freeman Dyson, a Princeton University physicist and a contemporary of Einstein, observed that the human race seems to have 'a collective yearning for apocalyptic doom'. There always seems to be another end-of-the-world scenario facing us and we seem to delight in blaming ourselves for having created it – from 'acid rain' to 'global warming' to 'the coming new ice age'. What a huge arrogance we have. The Earth has survived for billions of years without us and now we truly believe that a single species, a few little human ants crawling about on its surface, can destroy an entire planet in just a few hundred years, not even the blink of an eye to Gaia? Or maybe we're just idle and our belief in our inevitable doom justifies us doing nothing to improve ourselves and the planet we live on? San Pedro is unimpressed by such lazy behavior and thinking. He demands more of us than that and confronts us with a simple question whenever we drink it (the most fundamental question of all, in fact, for every human being to answer): *Do you want to live or do you want to die?* This relates to our personal dramas and illnesses as well as planetary ones. *Which path do you want to walk down – the one of decline, negativity and (learned) hopelessness, or do you want to grab hold of life and wring every last drop of living from it?* To help us answer these questions, the spirit of the cactus shows us the beauty of the world and ourselves, and how 'we' and 'it' are one. The choice becomes clearer then and we can leave behind our fascinations with end-times and simply get on with our lives, living fully.

This new relationship with ourselves and our planet is a change in perception and an eye-opening change of mind; a recognition, if you like, that we have been duped into an apocalyptic, self-blaming relationship to a world that cannot be saved (and nor can we) – so why try? When we wake up and see it for what it is though, in all its wow-inducing beauty, that relationship changes and we are no longer the pawns in somebody else's end-game. These are the words of a few who have realized this truth during their ceremonies.[15]

Kane

I had chronic heartbreak that didn't subside, even after two years. I knew that something in my life wasn't right, but what I didn't know was that this heartbreak was just the tip of the iceberg. It was only a symptom of a much larger, deeper, problem. I drank San Pedro in the mountains [and] was given answers loud and clear. I was shown how for the past two years or longer I've been really cruel in the way I treated myself after my break-up. I learnt that the evil I was experiencing was none other than myself, or a part of myself that had been abused and was buried. This angry, violent, destructive part had been sitting in the background my whole life but I was not aware of it. My greatest lesson was to forgive and love myself. [Then] I met Mother Earth and suddenly realized that I've been standing on her my entire life. I felt ashamed and stupid for not knowing that she's always right there – but I also felt forgiven, like any mother would do for her child. I'd say that yes, there is an intelligence to San Pedro and it is closely tied in with the Earth. The experience I had will *never* leave me! San Pedro answers your questions. Clearly and without confusion or the need for interpretation. I understood what had happened with my relationship and was finally able to let go.

Jamie

I know now that the truth is love, always has been, and always will be [and] I now recognize the resolve asked of me: never compromise yourself to another; never compromise that inner core of fire and strength and self-knowing. Keep in sight yourself. Love and embrace; fully engage; give and receive; learn and grow...*this* is falling in love. Give yourself entirely. In truest love, there is no holding back. Know your path, your calling. Know what it is you must do and in whose service you must never falter. This is the ultimate realization of love: there is no suffering; there is only, ever, the pursuit of truth. The world will heal and be saved. It will know and live in love. Make it so in everything you do, in every act of good conscience. Make it so in every thought you think, in every bit of magick you invoke and gift to the world in heart and deed. Make it so wherever you are and whoever you are with; give yourself entirely. Make life a celebration with them.

Ethel

I was able to perceive a more subtle web of energy during the day and in the countryside where the energy of the mountains seemed a bit slower. When I rejoined my fellow travelers I could observe how our energies interacted and how connected we are to each other and to the physical world. With every encounter we exchange information and energy and we come away changed just a little bit. This realization made me aware of my influence on others and theirs on me and I became careful with my interactions, conscious of speaking only the truth and of keeping my intentions pure. I was also aware of the energy that other people and how it affected everyone. One friend came in enthused by the mountains and his enthusiasm sent ripples of excitement through the group, many of whom visited the mountain with him during our next San Pedro session.

In the words of George Bernard Shaw again: 'Life is no 'brief candle' to me. It is a sort of splendid torch which I have got hold of for a moment, and I want to make it burn as brightly as possible before handing it on to future generations.'

Forget your 'great calling'

Everyone seems to be looking for a 'purpose' these days. The new age books tell us we must have one and that this is the only way to integrity and happiness. This makes purpose and happiness sound like things that are 'over there' somewhere – on the next horizon, over the next mountain...

Our minds over-complicate things because *there is no mountain to climb*. We are already living our 'purpose' in every action we take. To know what it is simply observe what you do – and if you don't like it, do something else; take action instead of sitting at the feet of more gurus who will tell you how you're doing it 'wrong' and how you must follow *their* system and become more like them if you want to get it 'right'. What's wrong with just being you? Who else's opinion matters? Your life is between you and God.

Finding happiness is actually very simple: *do what makes you happy*. Paint a picture, read a book, go for a walk. The more you do the little things that make you happy, the more your life fills with happiness. It's not some great cosmic puzzle or 'spiritual warrior's quest', it's just doing the obvious. But more to the point, it's *doing*, not thinking about it, or worse still, worrying over nothing.

Accept who you are; love your illness

Do you want to live or do you want to die? This question keeps coming up because all illness, heartbreak, depression are a choice. If our pain really is so great we are entirely free to make the second choice, or we can make the first and be rid of it. But most people do not exercise their right to power and make either choice. Convinced by society that they are powerless and must give the management of their dis-eases and the control of their lives to 'experts' – doctors and scientists – they *become* powerless and resign themselves to their sickness while also rejecting it or seeing it as 'the enemy'. Then they flounder in the middle of those choices, not really living and not dying either, but surviving, medicated and complaining. Take action *for yourself* and be free of it.

There is also a third choice: to accept your illnesses as part of who you are and choose to live fully despite it; to take it with you on your journey and embrace it or to learn from it. It is the tension between opposites that causes pain – wanting what we can't have (or, rather, what we do not allow ourselves to have) or not wanting what we do have. Better, as Dina Glouberman advises in her book, *The Joy of Burnout*, to simply let go, stop fighting, and incorporate your illness into your life instead of making yourself a part of *its* existence.

When you are hopeless, give up hope
When you are humiliated, let go of pride and choose humility
When you are disillusioned, de-illusion
When you are holding on to what you know, let go and surrender to what is about to become

Be of service to others

Action, not concepts, thoughts and head-stuff, is what heals and facilitates change. If we allow it to, the mind will take over and loop, locking us up in the same old story and keeping us confined in who we've become. And we cannot *think* our way out of this problem; we cannot use a sick mind to cure a sick mind. *Action* gets us out of the loop and opens us up to new experiences.

One of my students lost her daughter to cancer some years ago, but to her the grief was as real as if it had happened just yesterday and she could barely say her daughter's name without crying. During one San Pedro ceremony, however, she realized that she was imprisoning herself and her daughter's spirit in this air of sadness and in so doing turning her daughter's life into a tragedy, which is not how she would have wanted to be remembered or how she was in life. To honor her daughter in a way she would have wanted instead, San Pedro taught this woman to use her knowledge of suffering to be of service to others who were also going through pain, and to do so as an act of gratitude for her daughter's life. From that moment on she abandoned her world of isolation and constant suffering and became a guide and an assistant to others, volunteering at my ceremonies and at La Gringa's events in Peru, where she became much-loved by participants, one of whom described her as '100 percent awesome'. Her life improved immeasurably and she made new friendships and rekindled relationships with family members who she hadn't spoken to in years.

> *Until you feel the need to help somebody you will not be Love.*
> *You will want to help some pieces of you.*
> *If you want to be Love you have to disappear.*
> *Only in this way can Love flow through you to where is*
> *needed*
> *And you will not interfere.*

Being Love means... being.

Valerio Caponetti

(2015 participant in ceremony)

You have no enemies; there is no struggle

Envidia (envy, jealousy) and mal d'ojo (the 'evil eye') are seen as real forces in the Andes, which can seriously harm others, as can words which contain energy and, used with bitterness, malice or spite, become poisonous darts full of toxins and vitriol. And, of course, since most people are unevolved, hypnotized by social conditioning, they find it hard to think for themselves and are, to be blunt, in many cases just plain stupid. Jealousies, rivalries and childish squabbling are commonplace, not only in Peru. You might find yourself on the receiving end of some of this too. But those who behave like this towards us only become 'enemies' if *we* define them as such. They only have power over us if we decide that we are powerless and choose to see *them* as stronger than us. The fact is that they're not. They can't be since we are all made of that same 'big bang' energy, all in equal measure. No-one has more actual power than anyone else and no-one, inherently or by 'divine right', has power over anyone.

San Pedro teaches us, in the words of the Tao, that 'True power *seems* weak' – and conversely that a show of power is symptomatic of inner weakness. Rather than giving in to the showy power of others, then, you can discover a lot about such people when you realize, as Ralph Waldo Emerson put it, that: '[A person's] opinion of the world is also a confession of character,' and in the words of Eric Hoffer: 'You can discover what your enemy fears most by observing the means he uses to frighten you.'

An example was an elderly woman (let's call her Maude) who, through her negativity and constant criticism of others, ended up losing a number of friends and supporters all in a single year. Instead of using this as a spur to consider *her own* behavior however, her 'opinion of the world' became that her friends had all suddenly 'gone mad' for leaving her – which is how she explained *their* behavior, behind their backs, to her remaining friends, continuing the judgments and poison that had led to her loss in the first place. Even though every one of her friends had independently had the same problems with this woman and her destructive games, dramas and gossip, it must all be *their* fault because she was so obviously superior to them.

The fact, however, was that Maude's life was itself touched by chaos and literal madness. She had a binge-drinking middle-aged son who behaved like a teenager, who still lived with his mother and was resistant to growing up and facing reality so he hid behind beer, a father with dementia, who she couldn't help, and a fanatical and hysterical sister who also loved drama and playing the 'blame game'. In these conditions her own fear, most likely, was of the madness of her world and of being seen as 'mad' herself (which is why she also needed to be 'right' and more 'clever' about everything than everyone else – and why she had lost her friends in the first place). Still refusing to see herself, however, she projected her instability onto others so she didn't have to look at her own issues or do anything to change them.

As Ernest Hemingway wrote (and San Pedro would agree): 'There is nothing noble in being superior to your fellow man; true nobility is being superior to your former self.' Life gives us perfect, and often very obvious and direct, opportunities to see who we have become and make positive changes so we can move on and become superior to our former selves, as in Maude's case. But there is always another, lazier and less useful option: to maintain our self-delusions by pretending that we are superior to those who are giving us these opportunities. We become complacent with our dramas then, regard ourselves as the centers of the universe, and choose the friendship of our problems to that of our genuine friends.

If we are saints, the kind response is not to fear people like this ('petty tyrants', as Castaneda called them) or allow their labels to stick so we define ourselves in their terms, but to pity them in *their* fear and sickness and treat them with compassion. Since most of us are not saints, however, the most practical solution is to simply walk away: to ignore them and not engage with their dramas. Which is exactly where Maude found herself.

In any case, the only 'enemies' we have are those we give our attention to and the only struggles we face are those we allow or create. Better to conserve our energies to get on with *our* lives instead of becoming bit players in the lives of the sick and the weak, in the understanding that these people have no real power and are beyond our help anyway because they are too afraid of themselves to accept our offers of healing.

> If you are willing to look at another person's behavior towards you as a reflection of their relationship with themselves rather than a statement about your value as a person then you will, over a period of time, cease to react at all.
> Yogi Bhajan

Healing begins by knowing your story, the myth you are allowing yourself to live by, then opening your heart and changing your mind

Forgive yourself and others – by which I mean, *let go of the past and its illusory 'issues' and 'dramas'* so you reclaim your power from them – then find a new and better story to live by.

San Pedro shows us that the origin of our suffering is the 'God-shaped hole' inside of us. We have forgotten who we are, where we come from, why we are here, and where we will return to: that *we are the God we are seeking*. And so we fill these holes with alcohol, sex, illnesses, gossip, soap operas, bodybuilding, kids, entanglements, repetitive disastrous relationships, or a thousand other addictions and obsessions; the distractions and stories we use to attempt to make sense of our lives and give us some meaning for being. When we accept that *we are Gods*, however, and start to act with power and responsibility, these holes fill themselves. There is no more need for games and suffering, which become trivial and pointless self-limitations in a world of vast possibility. We wake up and heal ourselves.

The Andean Shaman's View of Healing

Understanding the human condition like this is fundamental to Andean shamanism, which is sometimes called 'the path of heart' and is guided by the desire to find love, peace and beauty, balance and harmony in life moment-by-moment. The principles on which it is based, and which are incorporated into every San Pedro ceremony through the spirit of the plant and the intentions of the shaman are:

Munay

Not struggling to answer the 'big questions' (which may be truly unanswerable anyway since every answer simply provokes a new question) but doing 'the little things' with compassionate and loving intent, so that every day is infused with a sense of beauty and we can sleep peacefully at night in the knowledge that, as far as we were able and aware, we hurt no-one by our actions, including ourselves.

Yachay

Using informed wisdom in our choices and actions, which is greater and deeper than simple 'knowledge' and intellect. The former is provided by spirit, while the latter is a function of the limited rational mind, which is often led by ego, habit and shadow. Yachay is one of the gifts of San Pedro, which helps us understand the truths of our lives at a more soulful level and – if we choose – to live in faith, true power and beauty.

Llankay

Taking appropriate, wise, and positive actions in the world so we build a soul that is powerful and light. Because of this the world becomes a less fearful place for us all.

Kawsay

Respect for all of life in the awareness that we are connected, one, and part of a whole or, in the words of Henri Michaux, that, at our most fundamental level we are all just 'a passage in time'. Knowing this, we understand the fragility of our condition and the need for love and compassion, because whatever we do we do to ourselves.

Ayni

Perhaps the best-known and most important of Andean principles, ayni is a way of reciprocity, a form of giving without the desire to receive in return, but in the knowledge, nonetheless, that we will be rewarded for our actions as the energy they create continues to circulate so that we eventually receive in kind what we have given to others. Again in the words of Michaux, it is the realization that 'one is nothing but oneself' and at the same time we are everything: part of a shared life and a destiny we create. Or, as John Lennon wrote: 'In the end, the love you take is equal to the love you make.'

Types of Dis-Ease

According to curanderismo (Andean healing), then, disease is not just caused by physical processes but by social, psychological, emotional and spiritual factors too, which take on material form – often as a gift, to alert us to our condition and the nature of the 'God-shaped hole' inside of us. These are examples.

Bilis ('rage')

This arises from emotional causes and is common in people who

feel themselves wronged by another and so excluded from justice that they carry their anger like an energy which is strong enough to lead to stomach upsets, heartburn, acidity or ulcers if it is not released. The burning desire of such people is for the wrongs they have suffered to be recompensed and while they are not they feel it in their guts like an impotent or repressed anger at the wrongs that go unavenged. They do not understand or have faith that ayni (in this context a form of instant karma) has already taken care of things so that those who have hurt them have also suffered their own pain; that they are already living in the hell of a worldview that would cause them to hurt another human being in the first place. The sufferer wishes to enact a human vengeance on their enemy, not realizing that through the same principle of ayni they would hurt themselves even more by doing so. In a sense, then, bilis is a desire for control, an intrusion into the divine plan, and the solution to the illness is simply to let go; to forget the harm that was done or, better yet, to forgive it in the awareness that forgiveness is a healing action *for oneself.*

Empacho and pulsario

These are blockages of energy at the top of the stomach, which prevents its normal functions and can cause digestive disorders. Shamans describe them as crystallized pain, sorrow or anger. Although they are more frequently diagnosed in women and may also be related to hormonal imbalances, with symptoms including restlessness, anxiety and irritability, men can experience them too.

Mal aire

This literally means 'bad air', although it refers more to a 'bad atmosphere' surrounding an individual or family. Children are particularly at risk as they are more sensitive to moods and environments. It can result in colds, shaking and earaches, all of which may have a symbolic meaning as well as a physical

presence (earache, for example, might manifest from a desire not to hear what is being said to or around the child).

Envidia: envy or jealousy

Problems also arise from more social factors, such as when a neighbor desires what is yours or resents you for your success. Instead of working to achieve the same results for themselves, however, they direct an unhealthy energy towards you and this becomes a form of spirit intrusion, which works away at your soul. *Mal puesto* (hexing or cursing) and *mal d'ojo* (the evil eye: staring intently with the desire to harm) are related to envidia and can result in vomiting, diarrhea, fever, insomnia and depression on the part of the person who receives such an attack.

Mal suerte or saladera

A more spiritual problem can also arise, known as mal suerte: bad luck, where the sufferer's energy becomes so low or they become so disheartened that they cannot achieve anything positive. A related condition, more common in the Amazon, is *daño* ('harm'), a magical illness that may have been sent by a sorcerer working on behalf of a client, and is therefore serious. Its symptoms include pain, fatigue, problems with breathing and, over time, the appearance of tumors or other diseases that take physical forms in the body. Daño must be treated magically to remove the spiritual poison or *virote* – the 'evil thorn' or dart – which has been sent to the sufferer and, in Amazonian shamanism, return it to its source.

Susto

Susto is soul loss; a condition where we lose part of our spirit or our energy becomes so blocked and depleted that we no longer have access to our full power or to aspects of ourselves that we need for our well-being so we can get on with our lives. It may arise from shock, trauma, fear, abuse or injustice, and its symptoms include nervous disorders, feelings of panic, loss of appetite and energy, lack of trust in or engagement with the world, or a general malaise and decline, as if from a broken heart.

Jean-Pierre Chaumeil makes an interesting observation about illnesses like these in *Varieties of Amazonian Shamanism*.[16] In the jungle traditions of the ayahuasca shaman he says, diseases are more often diagnosed as having been sent to the sufferer by a neighbor or sorcerer (as in cases of daño). The cure normally involves removing the problem and returning its energy with full force to whoever sent it. In areas like the Andes where San Pedro is the medicine of choice, however, such approaches have become softened – in Chaumeil's view, 'moralized' – so that the healer is now more inclined to locate the source of suffering not wholly in the spirit world or with an external enemy, but within the patient himself.

This is congruent with the teachings of San Pedro that we must face ourselves and our responsibilities so that we find our salvation within, because that is where true healing lies. What San Pedro shows us, then, is that the imbalances that have led to our illnesses relate to some kind of moral or social transgression on our part as well. It is this that has, in some way, caused our problems or at least contributed to them through a chain of events that gave rise to a disease-causing energy. Even if the illness *has* been deliberately wished on us by an enemy, we as sufferers are not absolved of all responsibility for our pain but are part of the web of interactions that led to it. Mal puesto relates to a curse that may have been directed at us by a rival, for example, but the questions arise, even so: what have *we* done to draw attention to ourselves in this way? Why do *we* have enemies in the first place?

Mal aire is another example. Even though it is commonly diagnosed as arising from a bad atmosphere in a home, it is not an entirely spiritual problem in the sense that outside entities are wholly to blame, but also relates to the social and psychological make-up of the people who live in that household, because if they were happy and powerful they would not attract such an intrusive force. The onus is also on the patient, therefore, to identify and correct whatever he has been doing to weaken his spirit and put himself at risk. By taking some responsibility for his illness the sufferer also gives himself the power for healing.

It could be argued, in view of this, that San Pedro healing is more sophisticated than that of jungle medicines like ayahuasca. It does not involve just one cause and effect, for example, or one action and counteraction, but necessitates a deeper psychological and moral examination of our own motivations, behavior and underlying beliefs. In this way we come to understand the wider patterns of our interactions and the subtle flows of energy that are influencing our lives.

The San Pedro shaman, as well as being a plant alchemist and a practitioner of traditional medicine, therefore also becomes a sort of psychotherapist, confessor or priest who can help us see our patterns of behavior and how they fit into the wider universe, or to unveil our traumas and disconnections from the flows of love that is the true order of things.

The Shaman as Therapist

Asked if she considers 'psychotherapy' like this to be a tool of the modern curandera, Doris Rivera Lentz, another of Cusco's healers,[17] agrees that: 'I need to use psychology in my work. I show the patient that he is not the victim of sorcery but is creating the problem in his mind. Bringing it out is the first part of becoming well again.'

'So 'black magic', like mal puesto and mal ojo – hexing or cursing – does not really exist then?' I asked her.

'It is true that some people will take vengeance through black magic when they feel prejudiced or offended in some way,' she said. 'Because *they* are sick. When people think they have power and feel superior the ego can become very negative. The first thing I do is wake up the consciousness of the person who has been harmed and tell them that evil does not exist. You are inventing it. Neither good nor bad exists...we create the good and the bad.

'I recognize that the person may *feel* attacked [but] when someone falls ill it means they are weak and the curandera must speak positively and encourage them to shine light on it. Then they can create positive thoughts for themselves. People get ill [in other words] because they are not in equilibrium with themselves. Resentment, for example, causes cancer. Someone who is aggressive and violent is weakened in their heart, stomach and solar plexus: the *ñawi* or *naira*[18] where emotional attitudes are held. In the Andes people will frequently consider an aching stomach to have been caused by sorrow. People who do not have the freedom to express their feelings suffer from throat problems, and so on.

'How does healing, like that in a San Pedro ceremony, help them?' I wondered. 'What brings people finally to San Pedro?'

'Desperation [as in an illness or spiritual crisis] will show the necessity of love,' said Doris. 'We need to work daily to balance ourselves so the collective fear [of a lack of love or a distant God] will not infect us. Even if those around you are overcome, *you* must maintain your center. Individualism doesn't work and this [realization] will unite us in a shared future... [We must] come back to a new kind of community consciousness.'

Another of Cusco's healers, Don Eduardo, added a little more when I put a similar question to him: 'What matters is that people come back to equilibrium so they are more whole, more human, and they remember who they are. People who are balanced also know something of God. Huachuma provides answers because of its powers, but also because it leads us back to God and...[in] the surgery of God...everything is put right and our courses in life are corrected. Curanderos heal; sometimes we even cure... But huachuma is the remedy.'

Many shamans say the same thing: that they, as healers, are the agents or ambassadors of God, that they have a *don* or a healing gift, but that God is the real doctor and San Pedro is the way to find Him.

The huachumera La Gringa summarizes these themes and the actions of the plant with these words:

> San Pedro reconnects us to the Earth and helps us realize that there is no separation between us – you, me, the soil, the sky. We are one. To actually *experience* that is the most beautiful gift we can receive. And so San Pedro teaches us to live in harmony, and that compassion and understanding are the qualities of all true human beings. Through this it shows us how to love, respect and honor all things. It shows us, too, that we are children of the light – precious and special – and to see that light within us.

Each person's experience of San Pedro is unique, as we are all unique, and drinking it is therefore a personal journey of healing and your discovery of yourself and the universe. But there is one thing which is always true: the day you meet San Pedro is one you will never forget. It is a day that can change your life…always for the better.

A New Scientific Perspective on Teacher Plants

New research by mainstream institutions such as Baltimore's John Hopkins University of Medicine – surprisingly, perhaps – goes a long way to supporting these views. For years, beginning with the Nixon government in America and continuing through the Reagan's ridiculous 'War on Drugs', which created more suffering, more repression, more erosion of freedom and, paradoxically, more drug-taking than in the in previous years, there has been an embargo on research with psychedelics; for example, into their effectiveness at curing physical and mental problems such as Alzheimer's and depression. Thankfully, this embargo is starting to lift and researchers are reporting promising results.

A study covered by the Journal of Psychopharmacology, for example, found that 'taking psychedelic drugs does not result in impairment of mental health or an increased risk of depression' and 'there are no significant associations between lifetime use of psychedelics and increased likelihood of past year serious psychological distress, mental health treatment, suicidal thoughts, suicidal plans and suicide attempt, depression and anxiety.' In fact, 'People who experiment with psilocybin,' for example, 'report it as one of the most profound experiences they've had in their lives, even comparing it to the birth of their children.'

The other substances tested by John Hopkins were LSD and mescaline, the 'active ingredient' of San Pedro and, while the researchers summarized their findings with reference to psilo-cybin, the results were the same for all of these substances: 'We've known for several years now that the psychedelic compound psilocybin found in certain types of mushrooms can cause beneficial personality changes in an individual resulting in a more open personality, which is associated with imagination, art, feelings and general broad-mindedness.' According to the test results, as little as one mushroom can cause these positive personality changes for up to a year.

A more open personality is also associated with greater success in life, according to the scientist Dr Robin Carhart Harris. Far from 'destroying one's life', therefore, the evidence points to the enrichment and enhancement of people's lives from the use of substances such as mescaline and, by association, plants like peyote and San Pedro. As La Gringa said above: 'The day you meet San Pedro...can change your life...always for the better.' The scientific evidence supports this.[19]

The True Joy of Life

This is the true joy of life, the being used up for a purpose recognized by yourself as a mighty one; being a force of nature instead of a feverish, selfish little clod of ailments and grievances, complaining that the world will not devote itself to making you happy.

I am of the opinion that my life belongs to the community, and as long as I live, it is my privilege to do for it whatever I can. I want to be thoroughly used up when I die, for the harder I work, the more I live.

Life is no 'brief candle' to me. It is a sort of splendid torch which I have got hold of for a moment, and I want to make it burn as brightly as possible before handing it on to future generations.

George Bernard Shaw

Chapter 3

Cactus Creativity

'Learn to Think Outside of your Head'

You are the wave but you are also the ocean
Isaac Abrams, artist

Repressive drug laws, even for state-approved scientists and researchers, mean there are few studies on the uses and effects of psychedelics in healing, yet alone in the creative process. Most of what does exist was conducted in the 1960s and 1970s before these laws came into force. Pretty much all of this research shows, however, that psychedelics have a major, positive impact on the creativity.

In 1966, for example, results appeared from what Rick Strassman, in his essay, Creativity and Psychedelics, called 'the most well-executed and designed study to date'. Volunteers received extensive preparation and screening for explicitly-stated research on how psychedelics affect creativity. The results showed that even low to moderate doses of LSD and mescaline (found in San Pedro) enhanced creative problem-solving, according to subjective reports as well as objective assessments of the practical applicability of solutions that research subjects came up with. The study also showed a carry-over of enhanced creativity for some weeks afterwards.

In 1967, Stanley Krippner studied 91 artists who had had one or more psychedelic experiences. Among them were an award-winning filmmaker, a Guggenheim Fellow in poetry, and a recipient of Ford, Fulbright, and Rockefeller study grants in painting. Of the substances used, LSD was the most popular, followed by marijuana and DMT, but peyote (a relative of San

Pedro) and mescaline were also significant. The artists were asked if their psychedelic experiences had been pleasant. Ninety-one percent said yes. When they were asked: 'Have your psychedelic experiences influenced your art?' 91 percent again said yes. None of the group felt that their work had suffered as a result of their experience. Those who said that their art had been positively influenced mentioned a number of effects, the most frequent example being a new use of eidetic imagery. Fifty-four percent also said there had been a noticeable improvement in their technique (a greater use of color being cited most frequently). Fifty-two percent mentioned a change in their approach, such as the elimination of 'superficiality' and the discovery of a new depth to themselves as 'people and creators'. Some referred to their first psychedelic encounter as a 'peak experience' and a turning point in their lives. 'My dormant interest in music became an active one after a few sessions with peyote and DMT,' said one musician. Another reported that his experience 'caused me to enjoy the art of drawing for the first time in my life'.

The impact of psychedelics on one individual was illustrated in the case of the artist Isaac Abrams who, in an interview stated that: '[The] psychedelic experience has deeply influenced all aspects of my life. It was an experience of self-recognition... which opened my eyes to drawing and painting as the means of self-expression which I had always been seeking...many difficulties, personal and artistic, were resolved. When the personal difficulties were solved energy was released for the benefit of my art.' When he took mescaline, he said: 'It was beautiful.' His inner life opened and he thought that he might discover his 'life's mission', a new sense of meaning through art.

'The psychedelic experience ...has been one of turning on to the life process, to the dance of life with all of its motion and change,' he said, adding:

Before...my behavior was based on logical, rational and linear experience. Due to psychedelics I became influenced by experiences that were illogical, irrational and non-linear. But this too is a part of life. This aspect is needed if life is to become interrelated and harmonious. Psychedelic drugs give me a sense of harmony and beauty. For the first time in my life I can take pleasure in the beauty of a leaf; I can find meaning in the processes of nature. For me to paint an ugly picture would be a lie. It would be a violation of what I have learned through psychedelic experience. I have found that I can flow through my pen and brush; everything I do becomes a part of myself – an exchange of energy. The canvas becomes a part of my brain. With psychedelics you learn to think outside of your head... Psychedelic experience emphasizes the unity of things, the infinite dance. You are the wave but you are also the ocean.

'To invent something new,' said Krippner, 'one cannot be completely conditioned or imprinted. Perhaps it is this type of an individual – the person who will not be alarmed at what he perceives or conceptualizes during a psychedelic session – who can most benefit from these altered states of consciousness.'

San Pedro-Inspired Modern Artists

Two modern artists, one a painter and one a musician, wrote of their experiences with San Pedro in my book *Cactus of Mystery*, and how their ceremonies with the plant have inspired their work. David ('Slocum') Hewson is an internationally-known artist who lives in the rainforest near Iquitos, Peru. As well as portraits, which he sells worldwide, he produces altar pieces and frescos for churches in America and elsewhere that illustrate his interest in religious iconography and themes – but with a twist. His style has been described as 'modern Renaissance'. Inspired by the old masters and often including gold and water gilding in his portraits, murals and frescos, the twist comes from his incorporation of visionary experiences and his knowledge of plant medicines into his work. San Pedro has helped shape his views on life as well as his work.

Peter Sterling is a musician who is also inspired by San Pedro. His first album, *Harp Magic,* was nominated for the Naird Indie Award and in 2004 his CD *Harp Dreams* went to number one on the N.A.R. top-100 radio playlist, remaining there for eight weeks and making it the most played new age music CD in the United States, Canada and Europe. It was then nominated for album of the year. In his account below (and in his book, *Hearing The Angels Sing*) he reveals how San Pedro gave him the deepest healing of his life and removed sorrows and blockages so that his music, through a deeper connection to love and forgiveness, could flow more freely.

Inspiration for my art by David 'Slocum' Hewson[20]

By the fall of 2009 my traveling [art] exhibit had completed its North American tour and was on display in Cusco. My host there was a shaman who does weekly ceremonies from her home in the mountains just above the city. My first ceremony there gave me an overwhelming love of Mother Earth – I could see her breathing, a living being. An abundance flowed out, everything that nurtured me came from her. I deeply felt the connection with her, which was a splash of grace in comparison to what I had seen in my travels. In the late afternoon I went atop the Temple of the Moon to watch the sunset. I had recently started the practice of sun gazing and coming down from huachuma was the perfect time for it. I stared into the sun for the final five minutes before it reached the horizon, and as I watched it I went into trance. In this state I began to see very specific geometry emanating from the sun: a sacred geometry. With my bare feet planted on the Earth and the sun entering my eyes, I felt I was a plant myself, between Mother Earth and Father Sun, there was nothing separate; all existed together along with the planets, stars, moon, galaxies all being one. A difficult moment to put into words, but I felt totally present. Every cell in my body was connected to it all, no past, no future, just present. I was in rapture with the beauty. I thought it would be a lovely thing to paint.

Just before arriving in Cusco I'd been contacted by a hospital in the States enquiring about a possible commission. They wanted an artwork for the entrance of the hospital's heart centre wing. They sent me a handful of words and phrases for the subject matter of the piece, but none of them except 'nature' resonated with me. Having visions such as those in San Pedro or ayahuasca helps tremendously for translating images into visual art and so does a strong sentiment, but without the visuals it can be more challenging to execute. In this case I got a strong feeling of a woman emerging from the Earth who was the Earth or a part of it anyway. In the background she was framed by the thing that gives me most peace: sunsets. That image eventually became the basis for the hospital commission.

While in Cusco I got into the practice of *despachos*. This is a ritual that is done to show gratitude to the Earth and involves burying totemic objects in the ground. If the despacho also involves your personal wishes and intentions, it is burned instead. Later, four friends and I decided to take a trip to Amaru Muru outside of Juli on Lake Titicaca. Amaru Muru is an ancient portal carved into a massive rock that resembles a dragon's back surfacing from the Earth. It is said that if you leave all worldly attachments behind you can pass through the door to other dimensions. We decided to stay there and do a [despacho] ceremony.

My intent was clear: I was going to ask for guidance in making the commissioned hospital piece to create something that spoke of showing gratitude to Mother Earth, exactly what I experienced at the Temple of the Moon. We drank huachuma at nine o'clock and soon my friend Sampi was in full conversation, channeling all sorts of fascinating themes and theories. Normally I would jump right in with Sampi, but this time I was not drawn to conversation and kept to myself waiting for the proper moment to proceed with my despacho.

After about two hours I got up and went to the door and asked if I could do my despacho there. I had gathered the proper materials for the offering in Cusco – coca seeds, coca leaves, scallop shell, incense, and a beautiful hand-made alpaca cloth. I laid out the cloth on the inside base of the door and slowly began the process of infusing intent into every object, comprising every aspect of my making the artwork, including envisioning it complete and the feeling of what it would be like. I spent about an hour and a half blowing my intentions on every symbol, including a crystal I had carried in my pocket for years. I find this very powerful: to give away something you are very attached to and do it with love.

I wrapped up the offering and tied it with string then sat there in silence listening to Sampi ranting in full trance, ridding himself of demons in the near distance. It was the 21st of December and a full moon night and the light was fantastic... I went over to the [fire] and when the moment felt right I set the offering on fire and allowed the air to carry my wishes. We eventually went to sleep and awoke as the light came, without getting much sleep. Although I felt an unusual fullness within me I would not be aware of the full impact and power of the ceremony until a year later, when I was back in the States putting the final touches to the painting.

I returned to the Amazon to begin my studies for the piece. I did a sketch out of my head of the ceremony in Cusco and used that as a base. I had a few months to send a more refined sketch of the composition for the approval of the hospital officials who had commissioned it. From huachuma it was evident what to paint, but it was still a commission and the hospital had given me parameters. I scrapped the parameters, however, and went with the inspiration of the ceremony. I emailed them an image of the 2ft x 4ft drawing along with a breakdown of the meanings of the symbolism it contained. They approved the idea, were very pleased with it, and said it was exactly what they wanted. They even sent me a poem that one of the donors wrote from being inspired by seeing the drawing. They told me: 'Just do it, we love it,' and I was amazed at how easy it was.

I started on a 4ft x 8ft version of the image next, using numerous studies of landscapes, figures, serpents, gilded symbols and hummingbirds. I researched the sacred geometry I had seen around the sun as well and found that it actually exists and has a name: 12 golden ratio spirals with radials. I gave myself three months to complete the hospital piece. I set up my temporary studio and got to work. By the first month I had the panel etched and gilded and was ready to begin the painting.

I got into a rhythm taking care of odds and ends during the day, and then painting in the evening and through the night, finishing between 3am and dawn depending on my energy. Then I would sleep until noon and have a superfood smoothie and do it all again. As long as my nutrition was sufficient I did not lose inspiration, but there is a fine balance between inspiration and burning yourself out. I have 45 years' experience of going to extremes, but what I practiced here was a constant steady stream of inspiration. I motored through the first nine weeks of work.

It was not until the 21st of December rolled around again that I thought back to the despacho I had made at Amaru Muru exactly a year before. Over the last three weeks of work until the painting was finished I had been gobsmacked at where all my energy had come from, almost looking at the work and wondering how it had got there. There had been some challenging moments in it, but on the whole it turned out to be the most fluid, joyful piece I had ever created and there is no doubt that the spirit of huachuma was with me as I made it.

Meeting the Divine Mother by Peter Sterling

We arrived in Cusco and made our way to Casa De la Gringa, a quaint and funky hostel owned and run by La Gringa. Immediately my attention was drawn to a hand-painted sign with an image of a beautiful flowering cactus that said 'San Pedro journeys'. At first I was a bit surprised by this openness, but subsequently discovered that San Pedro and ayahuasca are both legal in Peru and ceremonies are advertised around many of the cities and towns. As I walked around and looked in the various rooms, to my surprise I saw a Paraguayan harp in the corner of the TV room! I took this as a very good sign and immediately felt at ease, as if angels were guiding my journey.

Our medicine experience was at another retreat owned by La Gringa in the hills above Cusco. This special hacienda is called the Mountain House and sits adjacent to the ancient Incan Temple of the Moon, an enigmatic ancient structure carved out of solid rock by ancient shamans, where elaborate ceremonies would be performed at the time of the full moon. It was the perfect place for us to discover the secret truths of our souls.

After about 30 or 40 minutes the medicine began to take effect and I noticed that the colors around me began to look more vibrant and intense as I gazed at the flowers and plants. I could also feel subtle changes in my perceptions as I looked at the plants and the blue sky above me with its wispy clouds that began to resemble animals, people, and angelic beings. San Pedro comes in waves that rise up in great swells that overtake you and carry you deeper and further with each passing set. A wave will come, rise to a crest of intensity, and then subside gently into a period of relative calm and ease. With each wave I would get more energized and activated. I felt the need to move some of this energy by walking, and so I ventured out into the open landscape to explore the Temple of the Moon and its surrounding valleys.

Visually I was overcome by the beauty of what my eyes were

seeing. There seemed to be light emanating from all the plants and emerald hillsides that surrounded me. It seemed to me that the vibrancy of the color was very rich in the ultraviolet spectrum of light frequencies, which were coming into my retina to the optic nerve and stimulating and awakening parts of my neocortex. I could feel my pupils dilating in order to take in more light, as if my eyes were feasting on a rich banquet of luminescence and iridescent Technicolor pulsations from the rocks, plants, grass, and hillsides as well as the cobalt blue sky overhead. It was like being in a psychedelic dreamscape.

I climbed a high rock outcrop that overlooked the valley. From there I had a commanding view of the Temple of the Moon with the 20,000 feet Andean peaks in the distance. It was breathtaking! I sat there in contemplation and experienced intensifying waves of euphoria, but I also began to struggle to catch my breath.

Two days before I left for Peru I had contracted a respiratory infection with the symptoms of a raspy cough and runny nose and I had been struggling with my breathing ever since I arrived in Cusco. Now as I sat on my eagle's perch my symptoms began to intensify and my breathing became more rapid and difficult. To compound this I started to feel my heart race as I became overcome with anxiety from my shortness of breath. Over the years I have had various episodes with my heart and I wondered now if perhaps I would have a heart attack. I decided at that point that it might be wise for me to make my way back to the Mountain House. I did not want to be alone in case I went into some sort of critical situation.

I immediately went to La Gringa and told her my predicament and she fetched some cans of oxygen that she kept for emergencies like this. As I inhaled I immediately felt a relief and my breathing began to stabilize. I started to have memories of childhood. I remembered how when I was a small child, maybe five or six all the way up to my teenage years, my mother, who was a heavy smoker, would light up in the car with all the windows closed forcing me to breathe her smoke. I developed asthma when I was seven or eight due to this unfortunate situation. For years I struggled with my breathing, especially when I would exercise. My parents sent me to doctors who prescribed various inhalers that I would have to carry with me and use from time to time. Not once did my doctors or my parents consider that perhaps my symptoms were caused from breathing the exhaust from my mother's smoking. As these memories resurfaced now, I experienced an emotional release and I began to get angry and cry from the memory of my childhood struggle.

I told La Gringa that I felt like I was dying as I was overcome with more waves of anxiety and fear due to my problems in breathing and the potential I felt for a heart episode. She looked at me and smiled and said, 'Yes, perhaps you are dying!' I understood in that moment that this is the teaching of San Pedro. Perhaps I was meant to have just this transformational death experience. I surrendered to the increasing waves of anxiety and stress. I brought my hands to my heart in prayer and embraced the feeling of dying that continued to overtake me. Once again I felt the spirit of Pachamama holding me and I began to connect more deeply with the spirit of the Earth, with my own mother, and with all the past loves of my life.

I'd recently ended a three-year relationship and my heart was still tender from the end of our affair. I could feel an upwelling of emotion at this, connected to feelings of remorse for this ended love and every other ending over the years. I began to cry healing tears of deep release as I lay on the floor in fetal position. Even though it was painful to access this type of emotion it also felt incredibly healing. I realized I had not cried like this in many years and I embraced the opportunity to access the pain that was obviously stored within me.

After perhaps 15 or 20 minutes of this I looked up and saw La Gringa looking down at me with a gentle smile and eyes full of compassion and understanding. Sitting up, I asked if she would hold me. She said yes and I moved to the couch where I laid my head in her lap and began to sob more deeply than before, releasing the greatest pain that I have ever felt. This went on for perhaps an hour. Yet I was grateful for what was to be one of the deepest emotional healing experiences of my life. It was wonderful and liberating and healing at the deepest levels.

After a while my tears subsided and a feeling of deep peace overcame me. Thank God it was over. I felt cleansed, healed and renewed. It was like being reborn. I looked up with a feeling of gratitude for what had just transpired and happily said, 'Yay!' I thought the pain I had just released I would take to my grave, but that the alchemical combination of huachuma, the garden healing sanctuary, and the spiritual presence of Pachamama had all combined to facilitate one of the deepest healing experiences I'd ever had. I had waited many years for this moment, but now I knew that I was forever changed.

After a short period of time I collected myself and decided to take another walk out into the beautiful green countryside. Each step had the feeling of sacred presence and my soul seemed present in my body like never before. I felt extraordinarily and deeply connected to the Earth and sky and to all of God's creation. It radiated from my heart in all directions. It was like I had been awakened and rewoven into the very fabric of God through my newly-enlivened senses. How thankful I am for that healing and for the grace of God, the Divine Mother, and San Pedro.

Shamans as Artists

There has always been an affinity between art, music, and teacher plants, and the number of shamans who are also artists is remarkable in itself, so it is not too surprising that others, like David and Peter, have found healing and creative inspiration from San Pedro.

Probably the best known curandero-artist was Eduardo Calderon, from Tujillo in the north of Peru. Douglas Sharon, an anthropologist who worked with him in the 1970s, writes in his book, *Wizard of the Four Winds* about Calderon's initiation into shamanism:

'During my youth from more or less the age of seven or eight years I had some rare dreams,' Calderon says. 'I flew...and I went to strange places in the form of a spiral... I tried to restrain myself and I could not... I have seen things as if someone opens a door and the door is closed. I have had nightmares but not ordinary ones. I have seen myself introduced through a hole in the air and I went through an immense, immense world. I have felt numbness in all my body as if my hands were huge but I could not grasp. I could not hold up my hand.'

Sharon continues:

[Orthodox] Medicine seemed to be the best avenue of expression for Eduardo's idealism, but it was not economically feasible. His frustration, however, was temporarily mitigated by his growth as an artist...art provided the best medium of expression.

And so for Eduardo, his means for both making sense of and translating the messages of the spirits was art, a creative process he continued to work with for the rest of his life, even when he became one of Peru's most famous healers.

This, again, is not surprising as there is an obvious connection between visionary worlds and visionary expression. Shamans are sometimes known as 'walkers between worlds' and art is one way by which the intangible – the world of imagination and healing dreams – is brought into the tangible and the unseen realms become seen. It is fitting, too, that this process takes place through art. The information given to us by teacher plants tends to be revealed in a visual way (although not exclusively so; information may also be passed to us in an auditory or kinesthetic fashion or, especially with San Pedro, as a mood or a feeling: a 'knowing of truth') so it is logical that we would wish to represent the worlds we have been shown in the way that they have been shown to us.

How Art Heals: The Effect of Art on Consciousness

But there is more to it than this since art in itself is healing. Grant Eckert in his essay, Art and How it Benefits the Brain, writes that:

Art is very important in helping the brain reach its full potential... It introduces the brain to diverse cognitive skills that help us unravel intricate problems. Art activates the creative part of our brain – the part that works without words and can only express itself non-verbally. Art, in thought and through the creative processes, activates the imaginative and creative side, the spatial and intuitive side of our brain... It trains the brain to shift into thinking differently, broaching old problems in new ways.

This, too, is the nature of the entheogenic experience: it is non-rational and nonverbal, the insights coming at an almost cellular level through a remodeling of the self. Trying to capture this experience in words is too limiting for those who have undergone it. By splashing paint on paper, however, they put themselves back into connection with the experience and reengage with the creative process that took place then. Because they are no longer completely 'in' the experience, however, they can also glean more information from it as they record their sensations in art. They become, in a sense, walkers between worlds as well, not quite of this world and not fully in the psychedelic one that they have explored and re-emerged from.

Eckert continues:

> There have been copious studies on the relationship between
> art and its benefits to the brain...artistic expression is the key
> to comprehending ourselves...art and its expression [is] an
> expansion of brain function. In other words, art helps the
> brain in its search for knowledge.

When individuals create art and reflect on it, the process
increases self-awareness, awareness of others, and helps people
cope with stress and traumatic experiences. In many ways then,
artistic expression is the perfect adjunct to work with San Pedro,
which itself helps those who drink it to gain insight and
overcome stress-related health issues and traumas.

Most of us, however, have been trained by society to use more
of the left (rational) hemisphere of the brain, and like any muscle
used frequently it has grown in power and dominance while the
'muscle' of the right hemisphere – associated with the creative
imagination, serenity, synthesis and selflessness – has atrophied.
Music, art and other reflective techniques that lead us into a calm
and meditative state begin to correct this and bring us into
greater balance and fullness. We move from an everyday beta
brainwave pattern (where we are consciously alert or agitated,
tense or afraid) to an alpha pattern of physical and mental relaxation. By doing so we put ourselves in the ideal condition to
process, learn and retain new information. Relaxation is the state
we are in when we drink San Pedro and when we create art,
hence artistic expression is more than just a representation of the
entheogenic encounter; it *is* that encounter relived, even if our
work on the canvas bears no 'actual' similarity to what we saw or
experienced when we drank the cactus.

'It does not seem to be accidental that Eduardo the visionary
shaman is also an artist who sees shamanism as intimately

related to man's earliest artistic works and contends that 'without artistic creation in some form or another there is no shaman',' writes Sharon Lommel in *Shamanism: The Beginnings of Art.*

Calderon himself put it this way:

The power of artistic sensibility in curanderismo is...according to my evaluation, essential. In general the artist is sensitive, extremely sensitive...his expression is of a character which is not intellectual but spiritual. For this reason it goes without saying that within curanderismo artistic appreciations are essential...because the [healing] symbols [we see] are perceptible only to persons who really note a line, a trajectory of appreciation in order to be able to dominate the distinct phases of a curing scene... Those individuals always related art with mysticism, with the esoteric, with the mysteries.

The Impact of San Pedro on Modern Art

Even in modern Andean art – like the paintings sold on market stalls or peddled to tourists by street sellers – the influence of San Pedro can be felt, perhaps not in overtly 'spiritual' themes but certainly in the colors used by the artists. With San Pedro healing (particularly in its more modern form where ceremonies are held in daylight) color saturation is often a feature of the process. In *The Hummingbird's Journey to God* I wrote of one San Pedro journey where a simple marigold became so brilliantly bright that I couldn't look at it. This brilliance is referred to by several other participants in that book, and for some it is evidence of intelligence, sentience, and a living God-like quality to nature.

The author Aldous Huxley wrote of his mescaline experiences in *The Doors of Perception*, for example, that:

I was seeing what Adam had seen on the morning of his creation – the miracle, moment by moment, of naked existence...flowers shining with their own inner light and all but quivering under the pressure of the significance with which they were charged...a transience that was yet eternal life...the divine source of all existence... I continued to look at the flowers, and in their living light I seemed to detect the qualitative equivalent of breathing – but of a breathing without returns to a starting point, with no recurrent ebbs but only a repeated flow from beauty to heightened beauty, from deeper to ever deeper meaning.

It is this vibrancy and life that Andean artists capture in their work, using bright and contrasting colors to create a sense of this beautiful 'naked existence'. Simple everyday scenes are often the themes for their works – family gatherings, trips to market – the essence of 'transience' that is yet 'eternal life', for it is the simple things that San Pedro reminds us of: the beauty of love and friendship, the living nature of everything we see and are a part of, the wonder of life, and the sacred in the mundane. The remembrance of these qualities may also be partly where the healing arises from with San Pedro, bringing us a reconnection to the Earth, to ourselves, and to a God who is not distant from us and judgmental of our actions but ever-present, forgiving and loving within us.

Shamans as Musical Healers

It is not just in visual art, but also in poetry, music and song that San Pedro finds its expression in Andean shamanism. Many curanderos begin their ceremonies with a *tarjo*, for example – a 'power song', chant, oration or prayer that they sing (or have sung for them by their assistants) in order to purify themselves and create a connection between them and God before they start their healing or approach the mesa. This is the song used by Eduardo Calderon for this purpose:

I go along giving a good enchantment

A good remedy from my bench.[21]
Saint Cyprian
Who from the first years
With the three wise men
Cabbalist and surgeon
With my good San Pedro
All the potions
Of dead man's bones, ancients
Snake powder, antimony and minerals
Are all accounted
All the ailments of the entire body
All spiritual shocks, hypnotism, suggestions
Are all accounted
Saint Cyprian with rattle in hand
And his glass with the remedy
Well purified
He accounted in his great times
From the Huaringana I go playing.[22]
Curer, justifier
And at my game
Where beautiful Shimbe is accounted,[23]
Play!

In this tarjo Eduardo calls upon the powers of Saint Cyprian (lines 3-6), a primary ally and guardian, and refers to him as a 'cabbalist and surgeon'. According to history, Cyprian was born in Carthage to pagan parents who dedicated his childhood in service to the god Apollo. At the age of seven he was sent to apprentice with healers and magicians, and at the age of 15 he began his studies with the seven great sorcerers of his time, eventually becoming a magus himself. His practices included calling the spirits of the dead and bewitching people through the use of incantations and potions. In his writings he tells of calling demons and commanding them. His conversion to Christianity came in middle age, but he was always a controversial figure within the Church, and even today is regarded as the (unofficial) patron of sorcerers. What Eduardo is invoking here, therefore, is not just the saint, but his powers to summon helpful spirits and to control and banish demons in cases of spirit possession and exorcism.

In lines 7-11 Eduardo lists (and so 'brings to life') the healing tools of the mesa, beginning with San Pedro, then 'all the potions...dead man's bones...minerals,' and so on. The potions referred to are plant medicines, aguas, and other magical formulas for curing; the dead man's bones refer to the *huacas* (power places and objects) that may indeed be bones or cemetery dust, or some relic from a holy site which now have a place on his meas. The bones of the ancestors (especially if they were shamans or holy men) contain great power, and because they are taken from graveyards this power extends to interventions in matters of life and death. All of these, says Eduardo, are 'accounted'. That is, awakened by his chant and brought into play.

He next accounts for the body and its ailments, in effect claiming mastery over them. Finally (in lines 19-23), Eduardo talks of 'playing', a simple word that contains a number of meanings. Firstly, to play means to cure, but it also recognizes the fact that life itself is a play, a 'game', and that illness, in a sense, is a role we have chosen for ourselves. This corresponds to the Andean concept of life as a flow and exchange of energies, and the idea that as individuals we must take at least some responsibility for everything that happens to us as we are the ones who attract and connect to these flows of energy. As we saw earlier in reference to illnesses, for example, even in the case of a magical attack such as envidia where a rival is jealous of us and sends bad energies our way to deliberately harm us, we must ask ourselves why. What have we done to deserve this? Perhaps we were not humble enough about our good fortune and so invited the jealous attack?

Finally, the word 'play' is recognition that, no matter what may befall us, life is beautiful, an adventure, a game, and even in our most dreadful moments we must be aware of this because to take life too seriously is to invite ill-health, depression, and a diminution of the soul by becoming attached to particular states or outcomes instead of allowing the energy of life to just flow.

The Power of Song

Douglas Sharon, writing about Eduardo's tarjos, reported that he 'learns the traditional rhythms, but as with the various power objects [on his mesa] – positive and negative – he elaborates on the basic complex with his own particular talents and according to the inspiration he receives from a variety of extrapersonal and supernatural sources.' He 'freestyles' that, or channels new meanings according to his inspiration in the moment.

Calderon had tarjos for many purposes. To 'open an account' (begin a ceremony) for example: 'The invocation consists of chanting and whistling a special sacred tune (composed by the healer) to the accompaniment of his rattle.' To know whether a deceased person is in 'Heaven, Purgatory or Hell' another song is used. 'This is a special task, it is a special account and chant with which one looks in rarely encountered cases.' Even the ceremonial structure of Calderon's night-time rituals was divided by song. From 10pm to midnight there were prayers, rituals, and tarjos interspersed with whistling while San Pedro was drunk and its guardian spirits were called. From midnight to 6am – the curing part of the ceremony – each person present took a turn before the mesa while the curandero chanted a specific healing song in his or her name. Other tarjos were sung as particular artes (swords and staffs for example) were used to heal the patient, the shaman using song to summon the spirit of each. A final song closed the ceremony.

Sharon described Eduardo's practice as a 'modern' interpretation of traditional shamanism. His fieldwork, however, was carried out between 1970 and 1974, and things have moved on again in the intervening years. There are now even more modern interpretations to be found in the towns of the Sacred Valley, where shamans work with song and sound in a different way again. Chaska Lu, for example, is a healer from Aguas Calientes in the foothills of Machu Picchu, who uses a variety of traditional instruments as well as songs and chants to heal during San Pedro rituals. She calls her work 'sound healing' and offers this explanation for what she is doing.

> Sound breaks up energies. You have all seen opera singers who are able to shatter a glass with their voices and you know that ultrasound can be used in the treatment of cancer. This is similar to how we work with sound: to shatter and disrupt accumulations of negative energy which we see in the body of the patient or in his magnetic field [energy body].
>
> If there is a light energy [which I see as] like smoke or cobwebs in the patient I may use a horn to move it since a blast of air will usually disperse it. If it is denser and thicker, then a shrill whistle may be needed as a high-pitched sound will break it into a thousand pieces, like a pane of glass shattering. Throughout the day I also sing prayers for the patient since God is a musician and prefers the sound of beautiful song to dull requests, or I may chant or intone my healing into the patient. This is a form of prayer which finds its mark through song.

How Sound Heals

Shamanism is the archaic predecessor to many modern therapies and again, as with art and its documented positive effects on the psyche, it is no accident that music and song have long been incorporated into teacher plant ceremonies, not just as a means of guiding the journey and delivering healing, but also because it brings benefits in its own right. Psychologists who have made a study of the effect of music on the brain, on mood, and on healing have demonstrated some of these.

Research by Nayak, for example, shows that music therapy produces a decrease in anxiety and depression and an improved mood. It also has a positive effect on social and behavioral outcomes. In depressed adults, another psychologist, Hanser, was able to show an improvement in quality of life, a new sense of involvement with the environment, increased ability to express feelings, raised awareness and responsiveness, and new positive associations as a result of music therapy. Other research suggests that music can increase motivation and positive emotions even among those suffering from serious illnesses (stroke victims for example), and that when music therapy is used in conjunction with traditional treatments it improves success rates significantly, enabling patients to recover faster and better by increasing their positive emotions and motivation. Other research suggests that listening to some music (in this experiment, Mozart's piano sonata K448) can reduce the number of seizures in people with epilepsy. This has come to be called the 'Mozart Effect'.

San Pedro has the ability to amplify beauty – in the quality of music as it is heard as much as in art and nature – and a poignant or perfectly-timed song can shift the mood of a participant or steer a ceremony in a new direction or provide new insights and inspiration. It may well be that the first San Pedro shamans understood the beneficial effects of music on their patients, which studies like these are only now confirming in a modern clinical setting.

More Artists Speak

Let's end this chapter with the accounts of three other artists who have been inspired by San Pedro. Nicole Sky (known professionally as Sarab Deva) is a singer-songwriter previously signed to Sony/BMG Africa who was nominated twice in the South African Music Awards as Best Female Composer. After discovering plant medicine, Nicole turned her music towards mantras from a variety of Sanskrit lineages, with others channeled for healing and plant medicine ceremonies. Lydia Colón Perera is a painter who lives in the Sacred Valley near Cusco, and exhibits throughout Peru and internationally. Rik ThunderCrow is a Native American medicine man who has also maintained a dedicated Buddhist practice of chanting daily for more than 40 years. He sees no distinction between the use of San Pedro in healing and in creativity ('healing is a creative act; creative acts are healing') and remarks that:

> Huachuma and Peyote are an expedient means to open, amplify and expand perception, empathy and inspiration, leading to creative thought, motivation and courageous execution... These Sacraments have become my most valuable plant medicine and *Nam Myo Ho Renge Kyo* my most powerful chant to elevate the life-condition of the ceremony and its participants.

San Pedro healed my relationships with men by Nicole Sky (Sarab Deva)

Until you make the unconscious conscious, it will direct your life and you will call it fate
C G Jung

Fairly frequently in my life I have experienced the sting of unrequited love at the hands of what I would call a 'player' – the man you meet who makes you feel as though you are the only woman in the room and so incredibly special and beautiful, only to drop you as soon as you fall wildly in love with him. A couple of experiences of this nature left me feeling low in self-worth, a little broken to say the least, and years later still grappling with my inability to forgive those individuals for not loving me back. This wound went so deep that upon discovering yoga and the Vedic stories of Krishna I even struggled with the idea of people worshiping what I considered a dead-ringer for a player! Krishna! I mean seriously! He cavorted with all the milkmaids and had no sense of responsibility, quite the opposite of Rama who was the perfect father, perfect son, perfect king and perfect husband!

It was not until I drank San Pedro that I started to process this within myself and to understand the role of the 'player' in my life and in the spiritual world. San Pedro, which I felt to be a male energy, taught me to truly see the beauty in all things, even myself. I began to recognize the metaphor of Krishna, the playful aspect of divine masculine energy and His purity of interaction with the divine feminine. I grew to love and trust the Krishna-like carefree attitude and how San Pedro was teaching me to be less furiously focused on the outcomes of my life. I was able to translate San Pedro's teaching into my own experiences, clearly perceiving that just as the Moon (female) is unable to see herself in all her beauty without the light of the Sun (male) to shine on her, so those 'players' that I encountered were loving me and giving me perspective on my beauty when I was unable to do it for myself. I was inspired by San Pedro to start working with a mantra that relates to Krishna and the love of his mother after this healing: *Gopala, gopala, devaki nandana Gopala*. And through this I was able to transmute my resentment into unconditional love.

This is the song that resulted: https://soundcloud.com/nicole-sky-2/songs-for-san-pedro-gopala.[24]

We rarely hear the inward music
But we're all dancing to it nevertheless
Rumi

Meeting the mountain spirits by Lydia Colón Perera

I first visited Peru in 1997 and returned a year later to make Cusco my home. Shortly after settling here I attended a night-time ceremony with San Pedro at the Temple of the Moon, led by a shaman from the north of Peru. We drank the medicine around a campfire and some of us went into the temple. For hours I lay in a fetal position on one of the carved stone seats there, experiencing what I believe were journeys of past lives. I found myself as a 14-year-old Inca boy, then I became a wise old sage with a long white beard standing under the light of the opening at the top of the temple cave. The light reminded me of a white dove or the Holy Spirit, for it was a pure white moon that shone through the hole.

What I remembered most after the journey was that I saw Mother Earth being born and when the water broke it became Lake Titicaca. It all came together in a painting I did on satin, embellished with topaz and amethyst: *The Birth of the Earth*.

On another occasion, one early morning while I was watching the sunrise, I experienced a vision of the words 'Marka Wasi'[25] carved in a huge stone. At the same time I heard a God-like, booming voice say the name Marka Wasi. It was a call and I knew it, but what I did not know was that it was also another call from Grandfather San Pedro. That year I had the opportunity to journey to Marka Wasi during the full moon of August. On the second night we drank San Pedro and it became for me a journey to the stars.

During the ceremony I was asked by the shaman: 'Lydia, what did you come here for?' I told him I came to meet the mountains spirits. He spun me around and told me to look at the mountain in front of me. I found myself feeling very tiny and facing what appeared to be a giant bald eagle with a serpent in its talons. They were 'One', together in one *apu*.[26] That night the stars were connected with web-like streams of light that created the constellations. There were ships in the night that blinked with emerald, ruby and sapphire lights. One of my friends on the journey appeared to me as a beautiful Hopi maiden sitting under the Marka Wasi sky saying prayers to the mountains and the heavens. I again became a young Inca boy and played with a wolf while I sang in the light of the full moon. My prayer was heard. Not only did I meet the mountain spirits that night but I was also gifted with an inspiration from San Pedro for my painting *Hopi en Marka Wasi*.[27] This painting was shown in Cusco in November 2015 at an exhibition organized by the Ministry of Culture.

Thank you San Pedro for your continuing inspirations.

Creative healing through poetry and vision
by Rik Thundercrow

One day in 2011 the phone rings and I answer to hear that a family member has just been diagnosed with cancer. It's the kind of news that stops time as millions of feelings encircled by a rush of endorphins and fragmented cognition struggle for balance. A 'disturbance in the Force' as it were. A request for a Healing Prayer is made, but I knew this would become a ceremony more than a prayer because of the seriousness of the situation, and that I was going to have to dig deep within myself to free my entire being from the doubt, fear and the inner diatribe of logic that are obstacles to the Gates of Wisdom, Knowledge, Compassion and Enlightenment. I was going to have to challenge myself in a deep scary way – scary because one may have to face oneself in the unfiltered raw perspective of how the Universe sees you, just to present any prayer or request.

I prepared for a solo chanting, singing and drumming Prayer Ceremony and made an altar in the old Beauty Way, polished off with my unique signature developed over the years. I would perform the ceremony while consuming huachúma for two days straight, then right before falling asleep, I would play pre-selected music of a non-commercial, ambient nature and consume a final large dose of huachúma to enter the bardo of dreams.

I am within an enormous golden structured and delicately jeweled grand edifice of perpetually kinetic filigree of refined detail and color and beauty beyond description, suspended within repetitions of itself like Russian dolls – a presence of great beauty and compassion that occupies every direction, recognizes me by my prayers for those suffering, and by the prayers of others on my behalf which have guided me here. 'What is it that you have to offer?' I am asked and before I have the ability to think, my heart proclaims its true intent: 'With good intentions, I have thoughts, words, deeds and actions based on libraries of wisdom, knowledge, compassion and aspirations for enlightenment to heal all beings and end all sufferings.'

I suddenly awaken and experience the grand edifice mapped onto the real objects and spaces in my room – both realities existing in the same time-space domain – and I realize that I too am conscious on both sides of these phenomena! Things get even trippier as from the 'other' domain 'I' turn to 'myself' in this domain and request that I start a new note on my tablet, which I always keep at the ready for such events. 'Title this declaration *The Beauty Way Bodhisattva Prayer.*' I am instructed to write down every word as dictated, with no alterations! I am further instructed to perform another ceremony – 'Only this time do it with spirit to understand its core message from within your eternal essence.' After the dictation and writing I am promised that I will have another vision during that next ceremony and that I should 'have the writing tools ready for dictation'.

When I awaken hours later, rested and refreshed, I review for the first time what was dictated and what I have written on my tablet, and there it was! *The Beauty Way Bodhisattva Prayer* – a rather extensively metaphoric declarative prose poem. I'm not a person that makes the structured focused effort and goal to create something like that. My mind would be judging and analyzing the whole work into options and scenarios and obscuring any potential for creative flow.

I prepare and perform the next ceremony as directed, but this time it only took 24 hours. I fell asleep to the same procedure as last – consume a large dose of huachúma, smoke a prayer with tobacco/herb mix then retire with music, and this time with *The Beauty Way Bodhisattva Prayer* also in my heart.

Beautiful music drives the forms of an amazing vista of time, connected and meticulously woven and maintained in the domains of all directions, from the infinite past to the present and infinite future by Grandmother Na'ashjéíí Asdzáá or Spider Woman who pauses and swiftly pivots at the awareness of my presence! The projected gaze of her six eyes race through my optic nerve into my mind and down my spine, scanning and rendering a live image of my own working nervous system! That task completed, she relaxes from her protective demeanor and sends an extreme pulse through our connection.

What I was shown and experienced in that vision can best be conveyed by the following *Vision Poem* which was dictated during my journey and written down by me as per the prior stated procedure:

I've run the many prairies...
On many worlds,
In many forms...
Through many ages
In search of YOU!
Traversing The Mystery...
Swiftly – faster
And
Ever-further!
Until Now...
I've caught up to you,
We've met...
Yet again!
But I'm a prairie runner
And

I must soar the prairies a-new,
On new worlds...
In new times!
Lost and low for me,
To be...
In any time
On any world
Not with you!
We've run the many prairies...
On many worlds, in many forms,
Through many ages...
To find us!
Spirits danced
In our wake!
Come...
Soar with me!
We are magic together
Because
You're a prairie runner too
(September 2, 2011, 1:46am)

I was instructed to share both of these poems – *The Beauty Way Bodhisattva Prayer* and the *Vision Poem* – with my patient, who would then be cured and protected as proof of the validity of the visions and poems still in use among my people for healing to this day. I did so and am happy to report that the patient *was* cured through a holistic combination of inspiration from Huachúma, prayer, song, vision, traditional healthy practices and a good physician all working towards the same goal. So this is why I cannot see how a breakthrough in healing is not also rooted in creativity!

Now I am just being myself. I am perfectly imperfect, enjoying new creative collaborative projects in incubation stages. From the many, one will take flight at the right time, followed but the next, or something completely unexpected! I am driven by a vivid new awareness of who and what I am but more importantly, a deeper window of insight into the potential for healing we all possess through the utterance of a single phrase under the Sacred Light of Huachúma – San Pédro.

Chapter 4

Conclusions and Cautions

Working Responsibly with San Pedro

San Pedro shows us reality, but it also changes what we think of as real. I now understand our power, and that people have the ability to manifest anything if they choose. They just have to believe they can. San Pedro teaches us how to believe.

La Gringa, huachumera

In 2010 this comment was posted on the website dmt-nexus[28]: 'I was watching *The Nasca Lines in Peru* on TV and a shaman on that episode gave the host some San Pedro juice. The host (I think his name is Olly or Mark) says that it can be fatal if not prepared correctly. He said he was going to risk it in the hands of the shaman who prepared it.'

This is the problem with media 'experts' and presenters: they always want to build their parts up, introduce disingenuous drama to non-events and skew the truth to show the world how cool they are, especially with something like a San Pedro ceremony where there is not actually much to see on the outside except possibly a man lying in a hammock with a smile on his face. The transformation all takes place on the inside and that can't be filmed. And on the inside the only 'risk' the presenter is likely to face is one of ego (rather than literal) death, which I suspect that many celebrities would actually benefit from.

The reply that followed this comment identified the only real risk associated with San Pedro preparation and consumption: 'Anything can be fatal if you prepare it incorrectly. For example, when brewing San Pedro over an open fire, be sure not to stand *in* the fire. That is incorrect and dangerous.'

The website Erowid[29] makes the real situation clear:

There have been *no* verified human deaths from mescaline *ever*, although [the San Pedro cactus chronicler] K Trout states that there is one unconfirmed (and unconfirmable) report of a person who died during military experiments with the drug, after receiving a 15 gram dose intravenously (or about 150-200mg/kg). In experiments with rats, the LD50[30] for mescaline has been established in the range of 800-1,200mg/kg orally. Considering the human dose of mescaline is around 200-500mg orally, this means you would have to try very hard to take a fatal dose. It would be extremely unlikely to happen accidentally.

One unconfirmed death from a military drug experiment with mescaline versus the safe passage of thousands (millions?) of participants in San Pedro ceremonies dating back at least 3,500 years according to archaeological records sounds like pretty good odds to me that San Pedro is unlikely to do anyone any harm, and to do most people a lot of good (see the participant accounts in chapter 2 for some of the evidence). But these, of course, are not the media stories you are ever likely to read.

These figures are even more significant when you consider the number of fatalities each year from perfectly legal state-approved drugs. For example, alcohol:

Excessive alcohol use is a leading cause of preventable death. This dangerous behavior accounted for approximately 88,000 deaths per year from 2006-2010, and accounted for 1 in 10 deaths among working-age adults aged 20-64 years. Excessive alcohol use shortened the lives of those who died by about 30 years.
CDC[31]

Cigarettes:

Cigarette smoking causes about one of every five deaths in the United States each year. Cigarette smoking is estimated to cause…more than 480,000 deaths annually.
CDC[32]

And prescription medications:

The United States is in the midst of a prescription painkiller overdose epidemic. Since 1999, the amount of prescription painkillers prescribed and sold in the US has nearly quadrupled, yet there has not been an overall change in the amount of pain that Americans report. Overprescribing leads to more abuse and more overdose deaths. Every day, 44 people in the US die from overdose of prescription painkillers, and many more become addicted.
CDC[33]

In terms of anecdotal evidence, La Gringa tells the story of a young American traveler who broke into her garden and drank an entire bottle (about 10 strong doses) of San Pedro intended for ceremonial use that day.

The San Pedro flattened him and he lay on his back twitching and muttering about God for 24 hours, unable to move and with his eyes rolling back in his head. Then the next day he got up and apologized for his behavior, crying for forgiveness all the time. He left us a changed man and I don't believe he will ever act like that again.

Ten strong doses and he left enlightened, not dead.

In ceremonies with particularly 'stuck' individuals I have given some people four doses of San Pedro to get them through their blockages and there have been no ill-effects except for a few scratches on their knees from several hours of inspired prayer, thanking God for His blessings. The oldest person I have given San Pedro to was in her 70s. She joined the event with a friend in her 60s. Later, they wrote to me of their experiences:

> We appreciate the dynamic program you put together which has definitely changed our bodies and lives forever. We may be 66 and 72, but feel and look like 40 with your attention and help. San Pedro healed me in ways I never dreamt possible.

The youngest person to receive plant medicine from me was a fetus in the body of a pregnant participant. When the child (a boy) was born the doctors were concerned (as they frequently and unnecessarily seem to be with babies) that he might have a heart abnormality so they took x-rays, then called the mother into the room to show them to her because they couldn't believe what they were seeing. There was no defect, damage or problem, but there certainly was an abnormality: a pure white light radiating from his heart that had shown up on the x-ray; something they had never seen before. The child is now 10 and doing fine.

There are certain pre-existing physical conditions where caution with San Pedro is recommended, but overall and in general the risks from working with this plant are minimal to nil. These conditions include a bleeding colon, a severe heart problem and certain mental problems, especially if these have been treated by conventional doctors with anti-psychotic medications. Even so, there are instances of San Pedro curing all of these conditions under the guidance of a shaman in ceremony. The healer Valentin Hampejs says, for example, that he can cure schizophrenia in just three or four weeks with San Pedro and other medicines. At the website *Medicina Shamanica*[34] he says the following about mental diseases:

Psychiatrists only can describe the symptoms, they do not know anything about the reason of schizophrenia. But they think – as they do in the same terms with endogenous depression – that it is a metabolic disorder. And this is the only direction where they are searching and researching...but I know a little bit more. This chemical disorder is a consequence of a deeper disorder on an energetic level. It must have a cause. Any biochemical disorder must have a cause. It does not come by itself. But they think it must be the lack of a hormone, a lack of a transmitter substance or a surplus of a transmitter substance...they are looking just in this direction. But the biochemical disorders have a reason why they came to be.

[These diseases] belong to the darkness. Light is consciousness. Light is identifying with one's life and being thankful for one's life... This other side that belongs to the darkness must wait for a chance to enter into one's personality in order to get the opportunity to disintegrate it, because disintegration means darkness. Then you don't even know anymore who you are... Consequently, schizophrenia is a possession. Always!... These energies that enter are not neutral. They are energies that want to separate you from the light. Their intention is to possess you, so that you are theirs.

So how does Hampejs cure schizophrenia?

The chakras have to be activated so that the dark energy can be exorcised, with the help of the forces of the light of course. Through prayer, shamanic, mantric chanting and energetic cleansing instruments...you know the feathers and you know the blow with the medicine pipe and the blow with the medicine, which is made of fragrant herbs and you know the smoke and incenses...and also the help of all the invisible light beings which are around us.

The medicine [San Pedro] opens up the chakras, activates these energies, these demonic energies that cannot stand the light. What does Jesus say... 'Seek and ye shall find, ask and ye shall receive.' So, do you think that Jesus is a liar? That I can ask Him with all my heart for some blessings and he will not help me? And will not help me to help this person? We exorcise demons. And of course we do it with the help of Jesus, or with the help of some other representation of God. Of course we do it with God; and the Archangels, and Mother Mary, and Maria Lionza and all the shamanic spirits of our ancestors.

The medicine also helps the patient recall the primal trauma that brought about the possession.

You have to go through that, of course. This is part of the healing. The medicine takes you back. And you also have to be helped by the shaman in this process. You have to be stimulated, talked about. And the shaman is also given guidance...not only by the medicine, but by Jesus, the light spirits, by the sacred fire in our fire altar, by the nature energies around us, the elemental energies...we are talking about having taken San Pedro, the patient also.

So, once again, even with these tricky conditions, San Pedro can help.

Ceremonial Precautions

Despite the documented lack of ill-effects from taking San Pedro, there is still a big difference between conscious exploration and blind, dumb risk-taking; between taking sensible precautions and rushing headfirst into the unknown, so I want to suggest some precautions here, especially if this will be your first time with San Pedro.

Firstly, know what you're getting into. San Pedro is not a 'recreational drug'. It is a sacred *medicine*, capable of facilitating deep healing and a profound shift in consciousness *if* you approach it with clear intention and treat it with respect. If you choose not to...well, we get the San Pedro experience we deserve. So does that mean it's possible to have a 'bad trip' with San Pedro? Of course – because *we are* the bad trip! For years we have been carrying stale old stories with us that tell us we are wounded, damaged, unworthy and lost. These negative feelings are already in us, whether we are aware of them or not, and while we do not see them they are leaking out into all our relationships and creating our *mal suerte* (bad luck). That's *why* we're drinking the medicine: to see them and clear them.

So, while there is no 'bad trip molecule' in any teacher plant, the intention of all plants is to heal, and what we bring to the journey with us can determine how that healing proceeds. If we have come to the event thinking only that we will get high and screw around, we may be taken by surprise at the healing we get and, of course, we will then define it as negative and blame the plant. This is usually what people mean when they say they had a 'bad trip'. But if we come prepared and then relax and let go so the plant can do its work, the results are only ever beneficial.

Of course, the journey can still be challenging sometimes, depending on what we have hidden inside us or what we have consciously decided to face. But so can surgery to remove a tumor or five years of therapy to deal with a childhood trauma, and the benefit of San Pedro is that it can get it all done in one session and less painfully than the other options available. The plant may need to show us the reasons for our sicknesses, for example, so we can relive them, now from a grown-up position of power, and release them. It's not a 'bad trip', but a healing adventure and a cause for celebration when we get rid of the past and reconnect with the true nature of the world and ourselves, but that is why preparation is also important, why we should approach the ceremony respectfully and with awareness, and why we should give attention to *set* and *setting*.

Set

The term *set* refers to the state of mind with which you approach your encounter with any teacher plant. The most important practice for avoiding the unexpected and finding yourself face-to-face with a part of your unconscious that you are not yet ready to see is to set an intention for your journey. This provides a road map and a framework for the trip you are about to take. It gives it direction and purpose. Going into a journey without intention means that you could become overwhelmed, panicked and confused. Having a *reason* for taking the journey, however, means that everything you see, hear or feel relates to something definite and planned so you have some degree of control over it, a frame of reference so you can understand what's going on.

To set this intention it is useful to have a quiet time of meditation or reflection before you journey in order to clear your mind and focus on what you want to achieve. Shamanic plant work is not about getting high, but about getting results. Focus leads us.

Once your journey begins you may not always remember your intention as every question we answer for ourselves typically produces another, so some trips can be involved, depending on what you set out to explore. But clinging to intention during the journey is not so important anyway, as long as you had one at the start. In shamanic terms, intention alerts the plant spirit to your purpose so it is aware of the reason for your visit (like setting the agenda for a meeting), but we do not have to continually refer to it once the spirits have been informed, any more than we have to constantly restate the agenda during a meeting. We all know why we're here, so now we can just get on with it. It is after we return from the journey that we begin the work of understanding and integrating the information presented to us and this is when we refer to intention again. We can then interpret our experience within the framework we gave it so it makes sense to us and we have a plan for change.

Setting

Setting refers to the environment and circumstances in which San Pedro is taken. With any teacher plant, always ensure that it is taken in a safe, calm, quiet space, away from people who are non-participants, and away from noise and distractions. First and foremost, ensure that the environment around you is *safe*. It should also be supportive and conducive to the journey you're about to take. A tranquil, beautiful place in nature is better than a stuffy apartment with neighbors around. Have some blankets available so you can wrap yourself up if you wish. Light some incense if you want (palo santo is most often burned during ceremonies in the Andes). And if you'd like to play music, give some thought to your choice (it's probably best not to have a death metal band screaming about Satan at the same time you're meeting with God). Your journey will be a long one (sometimes 12 hours or more) so you need to prepare for it practically (rain clothes, sun hat, water and a torch maybe) and mentally.

Ceremony

The best way to work with San Pedro is in ceremony with a shaman who knows the medicine and understands what you're going through so he can help you if you need some support. If that is really not possible, at least have a sitter with you who has some experience with San Pedro and can help you practically and emotionally (if needed) during your journey.

If you wish to work shamanically with the plant you will also want to introduce a more formal ritual aspect. This will alert San Pedro to your intention to work with it and it also gives you a useful psychological boundary for your experience by providing the session with a definite beginning and end.

My procedure is to set up a mesa with *artes* – 'power objects', ritual artifacts and items of spiritual significance from sacred sites I have visited, each of which has some importance for me. I then make a prayer to the spirit of San Pedro and the other helpful spirits I wish to watch over the ceremony, and to the seven directions of east, south, west, north, above (Heaven, the sky), below (the Earth) and the centre where, symbolically, I will sit, so I am protected on all sides. I then seal the ceremonial space with a rattle to keep it pure and secure.

Following that, I drink the medicine and the ceremony begins at about 10am. If I am leading the ceremony for others, I call them together again at around 6pm to formally end the ritual and check on their progress. San Pedro will still be working in them for another several hours so we save the longer circle meeting until the following morning, then all participants have an opportunity to talk at length about their full experience. As this also shows, if you are planning a San Pedro ceremony of your own you should really allow 24 hours for the full experience (and probably another 24 for rest as it is unlikely that you will have managed to sleep much during the night).

Rituals gain more power when they are personalized, so you invest yourself in them, but this is a basic framework you could adopt for your own explorations.

Legalities of San Pedro

The legal situation regarding San Pedro is subject to change so it is wise to keep an eye on things yourself. At the time of writing, the situation is as clear and confused as it is with most other teacher plants. Clear in that the San Pedro cactus is perfectly legal to own and can be openly purchased and grown in most countries. Confused in that the mescaline it contains is regarded as a Class A/Schedule 1 drug. It rather depends, then, on the attitude of the authorities as to whether they might attempt to prosecute you for simply owning the plant. If you are known as an enthusiastic gardener and a 'cactus connoisseur', for example, you can expect to be left alone; if the police have an interest in you, however (for example, if you have previous drug convictions), it is feasible that they might try to tack 'mescaline possession' onto any other charge they decide to bring against you, at least as evidence of your character. It is worth noting, however, that recent attempts by police to bring convictions in Spain and Sweden for possession of kilograms of dried, powdered San Pedro, clearly with some suggestion that the powder is for consumption or supply, have both failed.

Erowid explains the situation with reference to US law, but this is pretty typical of the general state of affairs.

The legal status of mescaline-containing cacti is complex because the law is not clear. US Controlled Substance laws are unclear, confusing, and not based on any clear, rational criteria. San Pedro and the other columnar mescaline-containing cacti are *not* specifically scheduled, but they contain the controlled substance mescaline. Mescaline is a Schedule 1 substance in the US.

The wording of the Controlled Substance Act is that 'any material, compound, mixture, or preparation, which contains any quantity of [a Schedule I hallucinogenic substance]' is also a Schedule I substance. In practice [however], there are many common plants which contain measurable quantities of Schedule I substances like mescaline and DMT. While peyote (*Lophophora williamsii*) is specifically named in the law as a Schedule I substance, columnar cacti, like the San Pedro (*T. pachanoi*) and Peruvian Torch (*T. peruvianus*), are *not*. Since we are unaware of any convictions involving whole San Pedro and the case law contains no cases on point, it [therefore] makes their legal status unclear.

It is possible for a prosecutor to argue that it is illegal to possess or distribute San Pedro *with the knowledge* that it contains a controlled substance. This is based on somewhat analogous cases dealing with unscheduled plants like khat and mushrooms, but there aren't any exactly parallel cases. The main differences are that cacti are most often possessed as ornamental plants not for ingestion (unlike existing cases involving khat and mushrooms), they are widely available from legitimate retail outlets, and they are grown openly in arboretums and in gardens. In contrast, khat is listed in a Federal Register entry where the DEA says it considers khat a controlled substance container.

Please note: The fact that there have been few, if any, criminal convictions for the possession of San Pedro does not mean one is immune from police arrest for the sale or possession of these cacti.

We do know of one case where a person was prosecuted, and eventually pled guilty, for purchasing and distributing dried, powdered mescaline-containing *Trichocereus* cactus under an Illinois state law. Because the case did not go to trial [however] and there was no appellate-level decision, it is hard to extrapolate from this one prosecution. It stands as an important reminder that selling prepared mescaline-containing cacti products skirts the edge of the law and could easily be considered 'manufacturing' or 'distributing' a controlled substance. Practically speaking [however] it is very unlikely that someone would be convicted for simple possession of San Pedro.

There is a much higher risk to those who sell the plants with information about their psychoactive properties. Prosecutors are more likely to target sellers who advertise their cactus for 'getting high'. Preparing San Pedro for ingestion also makes it more likely that the plant would be considered a 'material, compound, mixture, or preparation' containing a Schedule I substance. There is little question under federal law about the legality of possessing or selling the cactus with the intent to use it as a source for mescaline.

These columnar mescaline-containing cacti are readily available from plant vendors across the country. They can be purchased at mega-chains such as Target and Home Depot and are cultivated on government properties and in arboretums. Because of this, simple possession with no intent to ingest is *de facto* legal. Cutting a propagable section (over 5 inches or 12cm) off of a live cactus would generally not count as preparation. However, slices, blended or boiled cactus material, pulp, extraction equipment, or any process of extraction could be considered preparation and immediately turns the plant material into a 'container' for a Schedule I substance.

The only case we know of is that of M Coblenz who was charged under California law for selling San Pedro. His lawyer defended the case by arguing selective prosecution. He was not convicted but we have no details about whether the defense succeeded, there was a plea agreement, or if some other circumstances resulted in the charges being dropped or dismissed.

As a side note, Richard Glen Boire of the Center for Cognitive Liberty and Ethics points out that it could be argued that the 'mescaline' that is a federally controlled substance refers only to synthetic and/or artificial mescaline. Because of the wording of Schedule I where peyote is scheduled by name, and because of the wording which specifically mentions chemicals 'of vegetable origin', it could be inferred that the explicit intent of the Controlled Substances Act is to not include substances 'of vegetable origin' in Schedule I unless specifically listed.

So there we have it. Pure mescaline is illegal; San Pedro (which contains mescaline) is not. It is therefore your action of removing one from the other (or your presumed intent to do so) that makes cactus possession illegal.

Of course one could, at this point, become outraged at the government's interference in your life and blatant attempt to control your cognitive processes and consciousness through the existence of laws like this at all. Whose mind is it anyway? And of what possible harm to others is a healing ceremony using a plant which has been regarded as sacred for thousands of years and could barely be used recreationally, which is attended by informed and consenting, supposedly-free adults with a right to choose for themselves?

One could also become disgusted at the state's money-motivated prejudices against plants like San Pedro, which have healed thousands of people from endless conditions and are more-or-less freely available to all (the real problem here, I suspect), while supporting drugs like alcohol, tobacco and prescription meds, which must collectively harm or kill millions of people each year.

Or one could just laugh at the sheer arrogance and stupidity of a 'God-fearing Christian nation' like America which at the same time declares that 'the all-powerful all-knowing God that we worship just plain got it wrong in His love for us when He gave us freely-available medicine plants. We need to suffer not heal, despite His original intentions.'

While all of these responses are justified – and all of them more logical and reasonable than the government's 'drug policies' and approach to teacher plants – under the current legal circumstances, it is probably better to just go quietly about your own business, gaining benefits from San Pedro but not evangelizing about it, campaigning for it, or raising your voice in any other way – unless you want your door kicked down one day on the flimsiest of legal grounds and the total absence of any moral grounds. As the huachumero Juan Navarro put it to me some years ago: 'San Pedro has a certain mystery to it.' Maybe it's best to leave it that way.

Final Words

As with all work in shamanism and with plant teachers in particular, it is impossible to simply read about the experiences of others and believe that we understand them or can apply the lessons of these teachers to our own lives. As the Salvia researcher, J D Arthur wrote in his book *Peopled Darkness*:

> Without some type of direct experience of the transformative nature of [these] substances...shedding light on the genuine fallacy of the validity of our normal perceptions and revealing hints about the true nature of the perceiver, any differentiation of the real from the false will remain in the realm of words alone.

The way to really *know* San Pedro is to go in search of its spirit yourself.

Appendix

The Three Fields (Campos) of the Mesa

Campo Ganadero (left of the mesa)

Literally, a *ganadero* is a cattle rancher, but the term is also a reference to 'one who wins or dominates' (from the verb *ganar*: to win). Its usage could therefore be associated historically with the oppressive power of the cattle-owning colonial overlord and the domination of the natives by the Spanish invaders. When contemporary healers are asked to explain the term they tend to correlate 'that which dominates' with Satan, and 'that which is dominated' with the human soul, which adds some credence, symbolically, to this explanation. The left of the mesa typically contains artes in the form of animals and natural objects, so 'herder' could also be taken to indicate the ability of the curer to control or manage 'animalistic' or primal forces.

Whichever explanation is most appropriate, this campo is always associated with negativity, evil, the underworld, manipulation, domination and black magic. A *brujo* (sorcerer) would therefore use this zone for *brujeria* (witchcraft), financial gain, enchantments, love magic and the control of others, while a healer needs it to help overcome these forces and to free a client from hexing, cursing or *mal suerte* (bad luck), since this field will reveal the sources of the manipulation acting against him. The magical number 13 is associated with this field, representing Jesus and the 12 disciples, the 13th of whom was Judas the betrayer.

Campo Justiciero (right of the mesa)

This is the field of 'the divine judge' and contains artes related to good (or white) magic. It is governed by Christ, who represents the centre of the mesa and is the lord of all three fields. The powers of this zone are concentrated in the central crucifix and in the staffs, which are placed upright in the ground behind the campo justiciero. The sacred number 12 (for the apostles and the signs of the zodiac) is associated with this field and the crucifix at the centre of the mesa is the ritual storage place for the *fuerza* ('force') of this number, as well as the seven 'justices', or miracles of Christ.

Campo Medio (centre of the mesa)

'The razor's edge'. The middle campo contains mediating artes in which the forces of good and evil are evenly balanced. The artifacts of this campo are symbolic of forces in nature and the world of man that can be used for good or evil depending on the intention of the individual, although the commitment to good on the part of the huachumero is shown by the fact that this is the largest field of the mesa. These opposing forces of the universe are not conceived of as irreconcilably in opposition but as complementary and necessary, for it is their interaction and the tension between them that creates and sustains all life.

This is also the zone that helps the curandero to concentrate his spiritual vision, which is activated and empowered by San Pedro, so that he can divine and cure. The campo medio is where 'the chiefs, the guardians, those who command, those who govern' present themselves, in the neutral field between two frontiers where a war can occur and territory must be defended. It is also therefore where the curandero must focus his attention and will so that everything remains controlled.

This campo is governed by San Cipriano (Saint Cyprian) whose powers are concentrated in the curandero's staffs. The sacred number 25 (12 for the campo justiciero plus 13 for the campo ganadero) is magically associated with this field. It is also the zone where patients' amulets and *seguros* are charged.

Seguro

Literally, the word seguro means 'insurance', 'assurance',

'safety', 'certainty' or 'protection'. In mesa shamanism seguros are herb-filled bottles which contain the healer's 'shadow-spirit' in the form of ritually prepared herbs and living plants which have a spirit that protects against *danos* (dangers such as curses, hexes and ill-will towards the owner of the seguro) while drawing in luck and good fortune.

A seguro consists of a clear glass bottle (often a rum or perfume bottle), which has not been in contact with garlic, onion or other strong seasonings. The herbs it contains will have been collected from enchanted locations, especially the sacred lagoons of Las Huaringas ('where the sky meets the earth'), as well as water from one or more of these lagoons, and perfumes, flower waters, honey, sugar, fragrant seeds, and possibly also small figurines, crystals or other miniature good luck charms. Sometimes the hair (and/or a picture) of the patient is also added.

The patient is instructed to blow into the bottle three times so that his 'shadow' is entrusted to the spirit powers of the seguro. By thus activating it, the patient has a permanent connection to the enchanted lagoons and the spirit of the plants, securing that person's soul to the power of these *encantos* (protective magical charms).

The patient receives the seguro from his healer as a medicine tool to be kept on his home altar, where it is considered the patient's 'friend' (Juan Navarro), 'second self', *nagual* or alter-ego. When it is brought back to ceremony the curandero is able to concentrate on it in spirit vision and it will show him the artes or healing actions most needed by the patient, as well as the causes of his dis-ease.

Endnotes

1. Stafford, P, *Psychedelics Encyclopedia*, Ronin Publishing, 1992
2. In *Sacred Plants of the San Pedro Cult*, Harvard University: Botanical Museum leaflets, 1983
3. Also see the Appendix for more information on the mesa layout.
4. Published by North Atlantic Books, 1999
5. www.erowid.com
6. One example of a 'true hallucination' was the discovery of the double helix structure of DNA by the Nobel Prize winner Francis Crick. Crick wrote that he was struggling to understand how DNA worked one day and entered what he called a 'dreaming state' (aided by LSD) while he had the problem on his mind. He dreamed of snakes writhing together and winding themselves like the serpents of the caduceus. It was 'a not insignificant thought', as he later put it – and from that true hallucination the problem of DNA was solved.
7. Aldous Huxley, *The Doors of Perception and Heaven and Hell*, Perennial; Reissue edition, 1990
8. https://www.erowid.org/search.php?q=san+pedro&fq= vault:%22CACTI%22&fq=section:%22PLANTS%22&fq=subt opic:%22preparation%22
9. See my books *Plant Spirit Shamanism* and *Drinking the Four Winds* for a description of other plants which might be added.
10. www.erowid.com
11. See my book *Drinking the Four Winds* for more information on tobacco.
12. In Ross Heaven, *The Hummingbird's Journey to God*
13. Isabel, Andean healer, quoted by Bonnie Glass-Coffin in her book, *The Gift of Life*.
14. *Paqo* is the correct name for a 'shaman' among the Qero

people of the High Andes.

15. For more, see my book *The Hummingbird's Journey to God*.

16. Jean-Pierre Chaumeil, *Varieties of Amazonian Shamanism. Shamans and Shamanisms: On the Threshold of the Next Millennium*, in *Diogenes*, Summer 1992, No. 158

17. Interviewed in *Plant Spirit Shamanism*, Ross Heaven, Destiny Books, 2006.

18. The Andean equivalent of the chakras. In the Quechua language it is ñawi, and in Aymara, naira. The words literally mean 'eye', but refer to energy centers in the body.

19. Story reported in Mint Press News. http://www.mint pressnews.com/from-psilocybin-to-mdma-researchers-are-in-the-throes-of-a-psychedelic-revival/210550/. Retrieved October 27, 2015.

20. David and Peter's accounts in this book are much-abridged versions of those which appear in *Cactus of Mystery*. For their full stories, please see this book, published by Inner Traditions.

21. Bench = the mesa.

22. Las Huaringas are the sacred lakes from where many curanderos take their power.

23. Shimbe are the sacred lagoons of the north, home to some of the most famous sorcerers in Peru.

24. This song was recorded specially for this book during a San Pedro ceremony in Cusco, Peru (November 2015) and is not yet available on any of Nicole's CDs.

25. Marka Wasi (known in Quechua as Wak'a Amaru Marka Wasi) is an archaeological site and a place of power close to Cusco (a *Wak'a* is a local god of protection or a sacred object or place). The site was probably the residence of Amaru Yupanki, the eldest son of Pachakutiq Inka Yupanki (1438–1471), the ninth ruler of the Inca state.

26. Apu = mountain spirit.

27. 'Hopi in Marka Wasi'.33. http://www.cdc.gov/drugover

dose/.

34. http://vhampejs.blogspot.pe/2011/07/shamanic-medicine
_26.html

MOON

BOOKS

Moon Books invites you to begin or deepen your encounter with
Paganism, in all its rich, creative, flourishing forms.